Dr Jonathan Swan's

QUACK™
MAGIC

THE DUBIOUS HISTORY OF
HEALTH FADS AND CURES

EBURY
PRESS

T5-CVH-152

First published 2003 by Ebury Press,
An imprint of Random House,
20 Vauxhall Bridge Road, London SW1V 2SA
www.randomhouse.co.uk

Random House Australia (Pty) Limited
20 Alfred Street, Milsons Point, Sydney,
New South Wales 2061, Australia

Random House New Zealand Limited
18 Poland Road, Glenfield, Auckland 10, New Zealand

Random House South Africa (Pty) Limited
Endulini, 5a Jubilee Road, Parktown 2193, South Africa

The Random House Group Limited Reg. No. 954009

www.randomhouse.co.uk

Printed and bound in Denmark by
Nørhaven Paperback A/S, Viborg

A CIP catalogue record for this book is available from
the British Library.

Cover designed by Gray318

All images courtesy of The Advertising Archives

ISBN 0 09188 809 3

CONTENTS

To Sharon and Esmé, for the consultations

'Nearly all men die of their medicines, not of their diseases.'
Molière

'The art of medicine consists in amusing the patient while nature cures the disease.'
Voltaire

'Be careful about reading health books. You may die of a misprint.'
Mark Twain

INTRODUCTION

What is a quack? One 1605 scribe described them thus: 'slow-bellied monks who have made excape from their cloisters, perjured shavelings, St John-lack Latins, thrasonical and unletterred chemists, shifting and outcast pettifoggers, sun-shunning night-birds and corner creepers, filthy graziers, cogging cavaliers, lazy clowns, dog-leeches and suchlike baggage'. This may provide a rough guide, but there's so much more to the world of quackery than deceitful con artists out to make a quick profit.

Ever since man first stumbled from his cave complaining that he didn't feel too well, there has been someone on hand to dispense medical advice. Some anthropologists think that doctoring may be the oldest profession, more ancient even than that other oldest profession. Cave paintings more than 15,000 years old have been discovered which show early medical practitioners in action – although they do seem to favour wearing antlers over a white coat and stethoscope.

There is some strange compulsion in people to give advice that seems to surface whenever illness or disease is around, a fertile breeding ground for quackish ideas and bizarre treatments. According to Greek historian Herodotus, the Ancient Babylonians took this to its logical extremes in their society. If anyone was unwell, he stood in the public square; passers-by were obliged by law to ask them of their symptoms, and, if they had heard of a similar case, or had themselves had the same complaint, they would be expected to give advice and treatment. Obviously this was a place for one type of quack to flourish: the enthusiast who recommends strange remedies based on their own, fervently held beliefs.

This type of quackery encompasses the whole gamut of medicine, from strange folk cures like rubbing snail juice in your eyes for blindness to pseudo-scientific beliefs peddled by people of learning, like John Cohausen in his 1743 work *Hermippus Recidivus*. There he detailed how it was possible to live to 115 in good health simply by inhaling the 'salubrious vapours' given off by the breath of young girls, recommending that men frequent orphanages and nurseries to avail themselves of the necessary exhalations. Even the monarchy considered itself a medical expert – King Henry VIII was the proud inventor of his own brand of anti-syphilitic plaster, made from powdered pearls and resin.

There is another type of quack, however, those who hawk their remedies with only one aim in mind: curing their own bank balance. Of course, these types have been around for centuries. The Romans had their fair share of quacks who sold useless potions for medical complaints, like turtle's blood ointment for impotence. But the golden age of quackery ran from the seventeenth to the nineteenth century. This was the boom era for patent medicines, when the lines between 'real' doctors and their quackish brethren began to be drawn more clearly (although plenty of people still worked both sides of the fence). Once famous products like Daffy's

Elixir, were sold throughout the eighteenth and nineteenth centuries as cure-alls, although Daffy's Elixir was of dubious restoratative ability, concocted as it was of brandy, with some rhubarb, aniseed and parsley.

Fraudulent charlatans, mountebanks, leeches or snake-oil salesmen have existed through every age of history, although they have changed their appearance to suit the times. Skull-caps and alchemical paraphernalia surrounded the seventeenth-century quack, whereas his nineteenth-century equivalent might appear top-hatted and suited, evidently a person of learning and 'quality'. Quack medicine could be just as much about appearance as anything else.

It's worth remembering, finally, that quacks occasionally have time on their side. After all, medical practices like homeopathy and osteopathy are more or less accepted as mainstream treatments now. Denounced as merely faddish and of no medical use at the outset, they have nonetheless pretty much seen off the tag of quack medicine. So remember today's quack could be tomorrow's far-sighted visionary. Dismiss them at your peril.

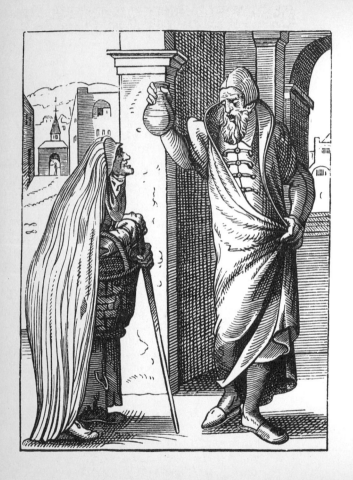

QUALIFIED DOCTORING

Every good doctor needs a reliable set of medical principles to guide their diagnosis and treatment of patients. This medical system, whatever it may be, provides the fundamental starting points for all diagnosis and treatment. How the body works, and what the physician believes to be the main factors in the cause of disease will determine the remedy. Some individualists have their own ideas, convinced for instance, that egg yolks cause all illness, or that jazz gives you cancer (as stated by Ruth Drown, twentieth-century quack queen). But other ideas have gained widespread acceptance, and, over the centuries, some established medical treatments have evolved from them.

The Four Humours

Not a Motown vocal quartet, but a doctrine that dominated medicine for over 1,000 years, the four humours were central to the historical understanding and treatment of disease,

Empedocles wasn't just a philosophical pioneer; he was also a man of fashion. Contemporary descriptions report crowds gathering around him, drawn as much by his flowing hair, laurel wreath, purple cloak and gold belt as by his oratory powers.

quack or otherwise. Initially it was Empedocles (500–430 BC) who argued that everything was created from the four elements – fire, water, earth and air – and each was associated with a particular characteristic – warmth, wetness, dryness and coldness.

From these elements and qualities came the idea of the four humours, which was adopted and developed by Hippocrates – yellow bile, black bile, blood and phlegm – each associated with their own temperament – choleric, melancholic, sanguine and phlegmatic. A balance of the four humours in the body meant that a person could enjoy perfect health, but an imbalance would result in illness and disease.

Hippocrates is commonly known as the father of medicine. Born in 459 BC, he gained such renown in his own life that when he died the honey made by the bees on his grave was thought to have magic properties. He pioneered clinical methods of observation and treatment, forsaking magic in favour of established and practised cures. His *Corpus* is a huge collection of writings about various diseases and illnesses (probably not all by him), and includes the Hippocratic Oath, the professional code of conduct that doctors still swear today. A distillation of his writings and medical knowledge are found in his well-known *Aphorisms*, which begins: 'Life is short, the art long-lived, the chance soon gone, experience deceptive and judgement difficult'.

Hippocratic followers believed that the body had a propensity to heal itself if left alone, and so concentrated on providing a supportive environment and diet to allow this to happen. If things looked really bad, then intervention might be necessary in the form of bleedings, sweatings and purgings to draw out the offending humours. The humoural theory also encompassed the four seasons: blood, the dominant humour, was like spring, warm and moist; yellow bile, hot and dry, was summer; black bile, cold and dry, autumn; and phlegm, like winter, was thought to be cold and moist. In time, the theory of the humours came to encompass the four tastes (yellow bile = bitter, black bile = sour, phlegm = salty, blood = sweet), the four main organs of the body, the four ages of man, and even, when the Christians got hold of it, the four evangelists.

Balancing the Bile

Once the theory of the humours was well established, doctors began to treat illness by making sure that the humours were balanced. If someone was unwell, it was because one of their four essential liquids was sloshing round in hazardous quantities and upsetting their *crasis* (the perfect equilibrium necessary for good health).

As this theory was elaborated by successive scholars, the idea of critical days was developed. When an illness was particularly severe, there would occur a moment of crisis, for example, on the fifth or seventh day. If encouragement or treatment was to be given, it should coincide with these days. Any treatment was aimed at restoring the humours to their correct proportions by drawing out the offending element. Favoured locations for expelling this *plethora*, or overabundance, was at each end of the digestive tract and out through the veins, and was achieved by the use of vomits, purges, sweatings and blisterings, and, most importantly, bleeding.

Vein Pursuits

Bloodletting, phlebotomy, venesection or just plain old bleeding has a long and noble tradition in the art of medicine. First amongst the so-called 'heroic' measures, it developed into an art in itself, with different schools of thought, methods and instruments. It was considered by most physicians to be the most potent weapon in their armoury against illness.

The Ancient Egyptians practised bleeding and thought that it went on in the animal kingdom – the hippo, they believed, bled itself by rubbing against sharp reeds. Hippocrates was in favour of the practice, although there was some opposition.

Blood was deemed the most vital of the humours, understood to be made from food. It also carried the vital spirit of the body, and as such was prized as a medicine in its own right. The blood of freshly slain gladiators was drunk in Ancient Rome to confer strength, and for centuries, blood was also considered a remedy for consumption. Insanity and weakness were often ascribed to blood deficiencies: one eighteenth-century physician reported an epileptic girl who drank the blood of a cat to cure herself. Unfortunately this remedy had disastrous side effects; she was observed to develop feline characteristics and spent her time howling, climbing on roofs and staring at a hole in the floor.

QUALIFIED DOCTORING

Claudius Galen, born in Persimmon in 129 AD, worked in Rome. His writings and teachings dominated Western medicine for centuries, and he had no small regard for his own abilities, especially compared with his contemporaries whom he generally considered fools. Doctor to the Emperor Marcus Aurelius, his reputation was secured by the Catholic Church who forbade challenges to his authority as his theories of anatomy dovetailed neatly with their own dogma of a natural system ordained by nature.

Another Greek physician Erasistratus (300–260 BC) thought it a dangerous practice because no one knew how much blood to take, and there was the danger that arteries and nerves could be accidentally sliced in the process. In extreme cases, he argued, how was bloodletting different from murder? Galen though, was a bloodletting enthusiast, and his views, which he expounded at great length, held sway until about the seventeenth century. Bleeding was, he declared, an effective way of evacuating *plethora*. Vomits, purges and starvation could also work, he said, but opening a vein was the quickest and most direct route.

There were two different methods for getting blood out of a patient: either a vein could be opened up – 'venesection' – or a cut could be made in the flesh and blood drawn from there, usually assisted by 'cupping'. For the first method the phlebotomist would use a lancet or fleam to cut directly into the vein, usually in the forearm or foot, and catch the spurting blood in a special bowl, which measured the amount drawn. In the second method devices like scarificators, cups and other suction devices were used to draw out the blood through punctures made in the flesh.

Generally, physicians believed in taking as much blood as they could, until the patient arrived at the point they called 'syncope'. In practice, this meant the loss of all sensation, and a faint and weak heartbeat. Doctors today would diagnose this as shock! One eleventh-century doctor believed that a man could be safely relieved of four-fifths of his blood.

What's the Bleeding Time?

The time when a patient should be bled and the duration of the operation was crucial. Medical calendars, almanacs, tables and wheel charts for bloodletting were published from the Middle Ages onwards, and avidly consulted by all involved in the trade. They depicted the signs of the zodiac, which related to the different parts of the body recommended for bleeding at different junctures of the planets.

By studying these charts a physician or barber-surgeon could be sure when to let blood and when to avoid breathing a vein. Roger Bacon, the thirteenth-century English philosopher, explained that bloodletting 'should be performed on a Saturday . . . on account of the malignity of Saturn who generates ill-fortune in all things'.

Bloodletting became so popular in England that by the end of the eighteenth century, people were bled as a way of maintaining good health. Spring and autumn were considered

By the end of the fourteenth century, many physicians were legally required to calculate the position of the moon before they carried out operations.

the best time to be cut open as a way of ensuring peak condition for the next six months.

The Professionals

Bloodletter, or the posher-sounding phlebotomist, was a proper profession that wasn't limited to specialist doctors. Barber-surgeons, who were in the business of pulling teeth, basic wound surgery, bone-setting and shaving, were also in the bleeding game. By the beginning of the thirteenth century they had organised themselves into a trade guild, and they carried on drawing blood at least until the end of the eighteenth century. Of course, 'real' doctors and surgeons could also draw blood, but their expensive fees meant lots of people relied on the local barber-surgeon for their corpuscle-draining needs. The red and white striped pole outside a gents barber today is a reminder that they used to do more than just cut hair and archive old editions of *What Car*. The stripes represent the red of the blood and the white of the tourniquet used to raise the vein, and the pole itself is the stick which patients gripped to promote the flow of blood. Finally, the ball on top represents the bowl in which the blood was caught.

In 1998 it was reported that bloodletting was still being practised in India for, amongst other things, arthritis and cancer. Patients flocked to Delhi to consult a phlebotomist who treated them for free. He required those who wanted to be bled to stand in the hot sun for half an hour before slicing their feet with a razor blade. Patients were adamant that the therapy had worked, one man claiming, 'After coming here, I have a lot of relief from my body ache. I don't take pills any more.'

Tools of the Trade

Anything sharp would do in early bloodletting days – thorns, stones, sticks and even fish-teeth were used by early doctors. But soon proper equipment was developed. *Phlebotomes*, sharpened lancets, were used by the Greeks (*phlebos* is Greek for vein), and they later became known as fleams in Europe. Practitioners of bloodletting had been advised since Hippocrates's time to carry different sizes of blades depending on the type of vein to be cut and amount of blood to be drawn, and various types of device were developed to help the surgeon get the blood out. Thumb lancets became very popular from the fifteenth century, small knives with adjustable blades of varying thickness and lengths, which surgeons carried around in decorative cases and pouches. The blood was collected in special bowls, which measured the amount taken.

Having a vein cut – 'breathed' – was a business best avoided by the squeamish. The site was chosen, with the veins in the forearm or foot most favoured. A tourniquet was applied to raise the vein and then the knife was quickly jabbed in. If the vein wasn't near the surface of the skin, the bloodletter would sometimes give the knife a wallop with a fleam mallet to knock it in!

Spring-loaded lancets were also sold, which had the advantage of making bleeding easy for those who weren't quite sure of their technique. All you had to do was line up the device over the blue lines under the skin, press a button, and a blade would automatically flick out and split the vein. One eighteenth-century American practitioner even wrote a poem dedicated to his spring-lancet, which included the line, 'I love thee, bloodstain'd, faithful friend!'

Medical legend has it that George Washington was bled to death by his doctors. He was suffering from a throat infection, and his physicians removed nine pints of blood within twenty-four hours.

The Cup Overfloweth

A different method of bleeding, which didn't involve slicing and puncturing veins, was that of scarification and cupping. Scarification was a way of obtaining blood by cutting through the skin and encouraging the wound to bleed, rather than opening up the main highways and byways of the circulatory system. Cupping encouraged the wound to bleed more heavily. Bloodletting experts agreed that specific sites were important for different ailments. Inflammations of the eye, for example, were to be treated by drawing off blood from the humeral (upper arm) vein on the affected side. This led to a great schism in medicine in the sixteenth century: some doctors believed that one should always draw blood from the same side of the body as the ailment, while others held that it should be taken from the opposite side. It was only the discovery that the blood actually circulated around the body in 1628 which ended this argument.

Nicholas Culpeper (1616–54), the English herbalist and physician, believed that a 'hot' liver, characterised by sweet spittle and red urine, could be cured by bleeding from the right arm. Ambroise Paré wrote in 1534 that the same arm should be opened to stop bleeding in the left nostril; the ankles of women should be cut to bring on menstruation; and the veins of the feverish should be opened to allow the heated blood to cool.

Professional cuppers were skilled people whose services were in great demand. An empty vessel, the cup, was drained of the air inside it, then clamped over the newly made incisions; the vacuum would effectively suck the blood into the cup. To empty the cup of air before it was applied, the cupper could extract it via a small valve, or use a burning piece of cloth, which was dropped in the cup immediately before being placed on the skin. The fire would consume all the air, creating enough of a vacuum to draw out the blood, although it frequently led to the patient being scorched into the bargain. A good cupper could juggle scarifying device, cups and fire all in a smooth sequence, and get the patient bleeding into the vessel before they had time to worry about whether it would hurt (which it did).

There were two types of cupping – wet and dry. Wet cupping meant cutting the patient's flesh and removing blood. In dry cupping, however, no incisions were made, and the vacuum cup was simply placed on the skin to attract the blood and humours away from the afflicted area. Effectively this was counter-irritation – pain in one area eliminated by discomfort in another.

Ancient Egyptian bloodletting cups made from animal horns have been found, and dry cupping has been used in Arabic and Chinese medicine for centuries. In 2001, a Syrian newspaper reported on the use of cupping in contemporary medicine. Conditions treated successfully by this method included heart disease, paralysis and gout. Adherents pointed out that the Prophet Muhammad himself recommended cupping as a useful medical treatment.

In cases of wet cupping where cuts in the flesh had to be made, the device most doctors favoured was a scarificator. This was a little machine, one which could inflict a number of

QUALIFIED DOCTORING

To clean a scarificator, the blades were sprung into mutton fat, ensuring hygiene for the cupper's next patient.

cuts simultaneously. Before their invention, around the beginning of the sixteenth century, people had to make each incision with a normal knife or fleam. A box of between twelve and twenty sharp blades were tensed and held in check by a spring-loaded mechanism. The box was placed on the flesh at the site from where the blood was to be drawn, the button was pushed and the blades would lash out, cutting a grid of small incisions over which the cup was quickly placed.

Scarificators and cupping sets became very elaborate pieces of kit. The blades of different models inflicted cuts in different patterns and could even make cuts, as the 1813 model did, in different directions. Decorated with ivory and silver latticework, the 'nasty little machines', as one doctor called them, were highly prized by practitioners. Similarly, cupping sets also became specialised, with finely blown glass cups in ostentatious presentation boxes available. Technology was also employed to make cupping methods more efficient. From the eighteenth century syringes were attached to draw out the air and increase blood flow, and rubber cups in the nineteenth century proved a great

Junod's Boot was the mother of all cupping devices. Rather than just cup a small area of the body, why not a full limb, wondered Monsieur Junod. In 1883 his patent arm and boot were registered. The devices were clamped and sealed on an arm or a leg, and the air removed, leaving the limb in a health-giving vacuum.

advance as they were less fragile and more easily manipulated than the glass versions.

Leeches

Although often used as an unflattering term for those in whom genuine medical skills do not reside as more than fleeting guests, the leech does in fact have a record of long and dedicated service to health. Its medical uses were noted by the Greeks, and Pliny recorded how they were used for gout in Roman times. For centuries they were used for all sorts of complaints, from restoring menstruation in sixteenth-century maidens to curing skin disease in the fourteenth century. Their golden age came in nineteenth-century France, when the craze for leeches was so widespread that ladies of fashion even wore dresses with leech-inspired prints on them. Swedish and German leeches were favoured by the medical profession as the most bloodthirsty, and they were bred on leech farms as well as being harvested from the wild in an effort to satisfy the demand. The application of leeches was favoured over cupping in some circumstances, particularly as they could be applied to sensitive areas of the body, such as in the mouth, around the eyes and on the sexual organs. One writer in 1550 even went so far as to recommend the use of a leech where questions of the marriage-bed arose. Young girls, who had misplaced their maidenhead before entering wedlock, could take advantage

'Leech' was the Anglo-Saxon name given to healers, and their trade was known as 'leechcraft'.

of the leech's appetite. By inserting a leech within their vagina before the wedding night, when their 'gallant husband' entered the 'citadel' the leech would be dislodged in a mess of blood and the illusion of virginity would be preserved.

Leeches were applied to the throat for tonsillitis, to the ears for earache and all over the body wherever they were required. Less skill was needed to apply leeches than was required for cupping, and they could extract blood more easily. To encourage leeches to suck continuously their tails would sometimes be cut off. What they sucked in one end just dribbled out the other. In the nineteenth century leeches were often applied to the anus to treat inflammations, and a thread was applied to their tails to stop them vanishing off into the body cavity.

Of course, man felt he could improve on nature and inventors began contemplating the possibility of constructing an artificial leech. These were really nothing more than vacuum machines. Holes were punctured in the skin (often in the same pattern as a leech bite) and then a cup, which was attached by a hose to a vacuum machine, was placed over them. Perhaps the most famous of these contraptions was Heurteloup's leech, which was sold in the nineteenth century. But the end of leeches, and of bleeding as a treatment in general, was already in sight by the time this device was on the market, and despite a last flourish in the mid-nineteenth century, bleeding in all its forms had pretty much died out altogether by the end of the century. However, the leech has made something of a comeback in the last forty years, mainly due to improved surgical techniques. Severed fingers, ears and other odds and ends have all been successfully reunited with their owners thanks to the humble *Hirudo medicinalis*. The gentle sucking action and powerful anti-coagulant chemicals in its saliva means that the leech is better than any man-made device when it comes to restoring circulation and getting rid of clots.

The Urge to Purge

After bleeding, vomits, purges and blisterings were the main remedies in any physician's medicine bag. If the body was felt to be overburdened with harmful material, then a spring-clean of the system was often the remedy of first resort. 'Regardless of whether this was the case, it was often thought prudent to empty the body of all removable material in preparation for a cure. Purges, or clysters, worked downwards; vomits and emetics upwards. Patients could expect to be purged or forced to drink emetics for almost any complaint: headaches, fever, bowel disorders, venereal disease, insanity and even deafness.

Hippocrates wrote that for someone suffering from fever, 'administer an emetic and clyster; and if these things do not loosen the bowels, purge with the boiled milk of asses'. The Egyptians also took great interest in their bowels. Herodotus (484–24 BC) noted that, 'the Egyptians use laxative three days in a row every month and care for their health through vomit inducers and enemas, because they are of the opinion that all human illnesses originate from enjoyed meals'. The excessive digestion that resulted from relishing meals would, they believed, lead to the food changing into harmful mucilaginous material, which would seep through the whole body, causing illness. Regular defecation was therefore essential to keeping healthy, and the top medical specialists of the time were the 'Shepherds of the Anus' who concentrated on this area.

The job of Shepherd of the Anus was important enough for the Pharaoh to have his own private one, who attended solely to the imperial digestive system. The Egyptians believed their faeces was laced with a highly dangerous substance called *wehedu*, which, while inert, could be absorbed into the body and cause all kinds of illness. Regular voiding was necessary to maintain good health and avoid dangerous accumulations. A common purge of the time was castor oil seeds chewed with beer, a combination guaranteed to produce spectacular results to this day.

A vomit and a purge often went hand in hand, as it was considered healthy to evacuate the stomach as well as the bowel. Any physician worth his salt would ponder the bile when it was brought forth, and would prescribe further treatments on this basis. As one eighteenth-century doctor and wit put it:

> For in ten words the whole Art is comprised;
> For some of the ten are always advised,
> Piss, Spew, and Spit,
> Perspiration and Sweat;
> Purge, Bleed, and Blister,
> Issues and Clyster . . .
> Most other specifics
> Have no visible effects,
> But the getting of fees,
> For a promise of ease.

Heavenly Medicine

Astrology has always been popular with medicine, and the stars certainly influenced physicians when they were diagnosing and treating diseases. The key idea was that the

A key idea when applying astrology to medical treatments was macrocosm and microcosm: the planets in the heavens (macro) affected everything in the universe, including the human body (micro). By observing these changes it was possible to divine what effect heavenly bodies would have on earthly ones.

planets of the universe somehow governed the internal workings of man, and astrologers drew up charts to enable medical students to divine the workings of the planets on the corporeal form. Inauspicious configurations in the heavens could lead to trouble on earth, as one seventeenth-century diarist noted: 'Taken with a strange Vertigo . . . with a sick fit in the Stomach like to vomit, which brought a sweat. The Moon opposite to the Ascendant in square to Saturn.'

The position of the planets dictated not only what illnesses were more likely, but also what cures should be administered. Temperaments and bodily disorders were associated with

Some physicians even believed that the stars had an influence on the potency of medicines. In the fifteenth century, doctors argued amongst themselves about the power of the planets on their pills; one argued that medicines prepared at the conjunction of Jupiter and Saturn worked best. Others believed that any illness depended on where the individual had been born – each city had its own planet, and treating disease successfully depended on observing that planetary conjunction. One doctor, Forli, a graduate of the famous medical school at Salerno in Italy, even declared that babies born in the eighth month could not live because that was when Saturn, who devoured children, reigned in the uterus.

particular zodiac signs, and horoscope analysis could help foretell a person's medical history and prognosis. According to a thirteenth-century astrology almanac, people born under Saturn's influence, for example, would suffer from 'long illness, particularly those occurring because of melancholy humours – leprosy, gout, cancer, fetid odours and bad breath from the mouth'.

Healthy people would have a general characteristic, for example, phlegmatic or sanguine, depending on the predominant humour in their body. It was important to recognise this when prescribing treatment, by carefully observing the astrological charts and matching the information with the patient. Woe betide the unhappy physician who treated a choleric patient, for example, when the heavens indicated it was the phlegmatic that they should be treating. The moon was the most significant planet in the medical universe. It ebbed and flowed the humours as it did the tides. Bleeding was regulated by the position of the moon in relation to the zodiac – it was thought that a patient should never be bled when the moon was in the same sign as the body part being drained.

This delightful remedy for dizziness from a German medicine book from 1596 shows how a spoonful of starcraft helped the medicine go down: 'Take a young swallow from her nest when the crescent moon is in Virgo; cut off the head and let the blood run into a vessel containing white frankincense; stir thoroughly until the fluid thickens; then give it to the patient when the moon is waning, three days in succession . . . see to it that the patient during the progress of the cure does not become angry.'

Strange Anatomy

'The stomach has the liver below it like a fire underneath a cauldron; and thus the stomach is like a kettle of food, the gall-bladder its cook, and the liver is the fire.' So ascertained a twelfth-century physician. The colon was widely held to be a sieve that strained faeces. The stomach was believed to be the central organ of the body, dry and cold and at the crossroads for all the veins and arteries. It was located at the lower end on the torso, reasoned physicians, because it was constantly churning and generating waste products; so far as they were concerned, the further away from the 'higher' organs and the mind, the better. Respiration took place because the intestines exhausted a gas, which was passed up into the lungs to be expelled. The Greek physician Galen spent a long time pondering the stomach and came to the conclusion that it was an animate creature in itself and that

One of the reasons for such odd anatomical beliefs in the ancient world was that no one had carried out detailed anatomical studies. Galen, whose anatomical writings held sway for about 1,000 years, didn't dissect human corpses; forbidden by law, he could only cut up animals (he was particularly fond of drowned monkeys), extrapolating his findings into the treatments he gave to wounded gladiators to whom he was employed to tend. Arab medical practitioners were explicitly forbidden dissection by the Koran. In the West, various medieval popes prohibited cutting up bodies, although this may have been more to stop the practice of boiling up the bodies of Christians who had died on the Crusades and sending the bones back for burial than to deliberately halt medical advances.

hunger pangs were a sort of existential angst, the result of an introspective stomach contemplating its own emptiness.

One of the key ideas of historical medicine and how the body as a machine actually worked evolved around the third century BC with the concept of *pneuma*, the breath and essence of life. This could be broken up into three distinct elements, which each had a different role. Animal spirit in the brain, the centre for the senses and movement; vital spirit, in and around the heart, which controlled body temperature; and natural spirit, which lived in the liver, the core of nutrition. *Pnuema* entered the body through the lungs, where it ran into the blood from the liver, picking up food from the intestines. The blood and *pneuma* then set off together for the heart, where upon arrival they loitered in the right-hand side while impurities were filtered out and expelled with the breath. The remaining blood then went through tiny pores into the other side of the heart where it was distributed around the body and brain, metamorphosing into animal spirit and distributed through the nerves, which were thought to be empty pipes.

Bizarre notions contributed to the misunderstanding of the human body. The Ancient Babylonians, for instance, believed that sheep were able to perceive the future in a way denied to humans. This knowledge was apparently reflected in the shape of their livers. The Hebrew Talmud catalogued the different bones of the body and arrived at the grand total of 248, including the celebrated bone of Luz. Situated somewhere between the coccyx and vertex, this bone was an incorruptible entity from which the rest of the body would be reconstructed at resurrection. Modern medical science has so far not been able to locate it.

Other strange ideas about the physical make-up and processes of the body held sway for centuries. The Greeks

QUACK MAGIC

In the seventeenth century, physicians were puzzled by the thyroid gland. Unable to agree on its purpose (or of any glands, for that matter), they decided that it was mainly of importance to the beauty of women inasmuch as it pleasingly filled out their necks.

had decreed that snot was the excrement of the brain, which ran out through the nostrils; it wasn't until the seventeenth century that this idea was effectively dismissed. It also took until the seventeenth century for William Harvey to point out that the blood circulated, and didn't move in tidal ebbs and flows, pulled by the wax and wane of the moon as had been thought previously. Ideas about how embryos grew weren't fully understood until Darwin, cell theory and the microtome. Until that point, some of the best theories had included: small mud babies, brought alive by the sun; tiny men (homunculi) held in the testicles and grown to life-size in the womb; babies being born only when they had mustered the strength to claw their way out.

A source of great frustration in the medical profession was the hunt for the soul. Greek medicine divided the soul into two: one part, the rational, lived in the brain, and controlled all the external and internal functions; the irrational lived in the

It was a commonly held medical belief that the soul would, if given the chance, always attempt to emigrate from the body if you sneezed. To combat this, a quick prayer or phrase would hold in the skittish soul (the origin, perhaps, of blessing sneezers).

Sneezing was also taken as a sign that the excessive humours were being expelled and the patient was on the road to recovery.

heart and the liver, and governed the emotions. Disorders such as madness and depression were caused by the soul being upset in the brain, or by illness in another part of the body having a knock-on effect.

The Egyptians would leave the heart undisturbed when mummifying bodies as this, their anatomy told them, was where the soul lived.

Medical School

Nothing encourages a patient to have faith in their medical practitioner more than a bulging portfolio of impressive-sounding qualifications and certificates. Any doctor can indulge his vanity and reassure his patients by adorning the walls of his office with degrees and licences that years of study have procured. Implicit faith in a doctor can, as Freud noted, have a beneficial effect on the health of patients before any treatment has even begun. But not all medical qualifications are so inspiring. Consider this medieval route of becoming a healer, taken from an English collection of folk cures:

> First get a toad. Take it to a graveyard and find a grave with an anthill on it. Bury the toad in the middle of the anthill, then return to the grave at midnight for the next three nights. On the fourth night, dig down into the anthill and you will find that the ants have eaten all the flesh of the toad, leaving only the bones. Take the bones and throw them into a stream. All the bones except one will flow away downstream, which will go against the current. Get hold of this bone; it . . . will give you special power.

Easier than years at medical school, but would it really inspire confidence? Of course, quacks have always claimed (and still do) medical qualifications they do not have, often inventing nonsense diplomas and testimonials to impress their clientele.

In the seventeenth century, quacks often masqueraded with foreign titles to add an air of professional mystique. 'High German' doctors abounded, who claimed their expertise in treating anything from the pox to the plague had been painstakingly gained in secret and exclusive European seats of learning. Some quacks, like the eighteenth-century oculist John Taylor, even spoke in a strange made-up language to impress the punters with their learning, which earned them the scorn of the educated classes who could tell the sound of babbled mumbo-jumbo when they heard it. Quacks had a field day in the USA where, until the late nineteenth century, anyone could call themselves doctor if they wanted to, regardless of whether they had received any tuition. Nonetheless, some still found it necessary to legitimise themselves with pieces of paper detailing their fraudulent credentials, and the supply of bogus medical certificates from 'diploma mills' is a business worth millions of dollars even today. A recent investigation in the US revealed that at least ninety-two doctors were practising in various hospitals with false qualifications.

Rather than relying on easily faked documentation, the Ancient Persians had a unique way of telling if someone was cut out for a career in medicine. According to the Vendidad, the Persian religious text, anyone wishing to become a doctor first had to prove themselves up to the job, in an early example of the three-strikes-and-you're-out rule. The budding medical student would experiment on unbelievers,

The Vendidad also specified a fee structure for medical treatment, which showed admirable principles. The clergy were treated for the price of a blessing, while the heads of a house, village or town had to pay the price of an ox, of low, average or high value respectively. A lord had to part with a chariot and four horses. Bizarrely, physicians also had to treat animals. Payment was in the form of the animal one hierarchical rung below the one treated; in the case of the sheep, the lowest animal on the list, the payment was the price of a good meal. Dogs, which were top of the pile, were to receive the same drugs as rich men. If the dog didn't want to take his medicine, it was acceptable for the physician to tie him up and force his mouth open with a stick.

and if a trio of patients died at his hands, he was branded incapable and forbidden to practise. However, if he managed to cure all three patients, he would be welcomed to the brotherhood of medicine and allowed to practise 'for ever and ever'.

Bedside Manners

A good bedside manner is an essential skill for any physician, and perhaps even more so for quacks. Patients are reassured by doctors who know, or appear to know, medical secrets beyond the reach of the layman. As the thirteenth-century *De Cautelis Medici* – 'Hints for Doctors' – advised, bluffing at the bedside was (and is) a legitimate tactic: 'Suppose you know nothing, say there is an obstruction of the liver,' it counselled. Awkward opinions from patients were easily dismissed: 'Perhaps he will reply, "Nay master, it is my head or legs (or other members) that trouble me." Repeat that it comes from the liver or stomach, and especially use the word obstruction, for patients do not understand it, which is very important.' To reassure patients that their money was being well spent it was vital to appear a practical man of science: 'When you go to a patient, always try to do something new every day, lest they say you are good at nothing but books.' And even when things didn't work out, remaining in control, or at least giving the appearance of unperturbed professionalism, was also vital, as the final piece of advice recognised: 'If you unfortunately visit a patient and find him dead, and they ask why you are come, say you knew he would die that night, but want to know at what hour he died.'

Quacks have always covered the tracks of their ignorance with well-chosen pseudoscientific jargon, or, failing that, relying on their authoritative manner to sway their patients. They didn't come much grander than the head of the Catholic Church. After all, who was going to argue with medical advice from God's representative on earth? This patently foolish remedy for female hysteria was recommended by Pope John XX, a man whose scriptural knowledge was unaccompanied by similar medical learning: 'A large cupping-glass be applied to the lower part of the patient's abdomen, with free use of the cautery, it will most thoroughly cure this disease. In hysterical fainting blow pepper and salt up the patient's nose. She will soon come round.'

Henri de Mondeville in the thirteenth century thought lying to his patients a good idea if it would help. Doctors could fake 'letters about the deaths of his enemies, or – if he is a spiritual man – by telling him that he has been made a bishop'.

Some patients are convinced of a quack's brilliance, despite all the evidence to the contrary. One such, a Signor Riminni, was arrested in Rome in 1997 for selling fake cough medicine, which was in fact nothing more than cabbage water. This didn't stop over 150 outraged citizens contacting the authorities, however, who all swore that his treatment had worked for them.

Of course, any patient would be convinced by a doctor who appeared to be in the pink of health. Here was a man, they would reason, whose own physical well-being was an advert for his skill, a belief exploited by many quacks. An Italian who made a quick buck in seventeenth-century England was Signor Winter. Shrewd enough to recognise that nothing advertised products as well as a doctor's own health, he claimed that he was a venerable ninety-eight years old, although he felt himself 'as strong as anyone of fifty'. The key to the youthful spring in his step was of course his own 'Elixir Vitae', invented by himself and apparently able to cure any disease, as well as confer longevity. Blended from sixty-two ingredients, it was imperative to keep a bottle close to hand, said the doctor. Winter claimed to carry a bottle round with him at all times, at night storing it under his pillow so that if at night, on finding himself, 'distempered, he taketh a spoonful or two'.

Diagnosis and Death

With such bizarre longstanding beliefs about the causes of illness, it was no wonder that strange methods of diagnosis came to the fore. Quacks, especially in the first half of the twentieth century, exploited this angle when they combined new technology not only with treating diseases, but also fraudulently 'discovering' them with their gadgetry (*see* Potions, Pills and Machines). But strange diagnostic methods have always been employed.

One particular brand of quacks were the 'pisse prophets' – doctors who gazed at, sniffed and even tasted the urine of patients to find out what ailed them. Water casting, or uroscopy, was a speciality that can be traced at least as far back as the thirteenth century. The textbook on the subject, *De Urinas*, told students that an understanding of the pulse and a careful study of urine were required to practise as a physician. A whole science grew up around urology, with charts illustrating the myriad complaints that could be detected from the sample of an ill patient. As urine casting fell out of favour with orthodox medicine, quacks moved in to fill a gap in the market. These 'pisse prophets' would often advertise themselves by hanging a pot or urinal outside their premises, and would diagnose the illness from the specimen provided, often without ever seeing the patient. One quack, working in seventeenth-century London, claimed he was able to tell in such detail the condition of a patient from their urine that he could even say with certainty how many stairs an injured man had fallen down when presented with his sample. It was not uncommon to send along one's servant with a sample of urine to the doctors, and for the servant to return later with necessary medicine for the complaint, which had been remotely diagnosed.

Looking for the causes of illness and disease led physicians and healers down some peculiar paths.

The Anglo-Saxons, for example, firmly believed in elf-shot as a reason for illness. Elves, they believed, unleashed volleys of tiny arrows, which pierced the body, causing illness.

QUALIFIED DOCTORING

Malicious and unpredictable, elves were understood to need no provoking in order to use someone as target practice.

Egyptian doctors often diagnosed illness as being blown into the body by a god or powerful magical entity, usually through the 'weaker' left side. Diseases of the heart and stomach, it was thought, were caused by 'poison seeds', implanted in the victims at night by malevolent spirits.

The idea of worms and serpents that lived in the body and caused ill health is an ancient one. These 'bosom serpents', often accompanied by their accomplice toads, frogs and lizards, were often blamed for causing stomach and intestinal disorders. It was believed that they entered the body either by slithering down the throat of unsuspecting sleepers, or were swallowed as spawn while the victim was drinking pond water. Medieval tales of patients who vomited snakes and toads at will were not uncommon, and doctors devised special cures for these patients – horse's urine could be drunk to flush them up, for example. You could also dangle a piece of bread baited on a hook down the patient's throat – the unwanted creature within would be unable to resist this morsel, and on taking a bite would be hauled out.

Worms were also diagnosed as the source of different illnesses. Toothache was, for centuries, believed to be the

 The *Daily Telegraph* ran a story in 1982 about a Syrian woman who reportedly had been taken to hospital with stomach pains. When doctors put a camera down her throat to see what was going on, they found themselves eyeball to eyeball with a six-foot snake, which had taken up residence there, squawking like a chicken whenever it was hungry. Apparently.

result of worms in the jaw. Diseases where worms and lice, teeming under the skin, were held to be causing cancers and ulcers were treated by suspending patients above vats of warm water to entice out the little critters.

It was always imperative that the ancient physicians diagnosed death correctly. Fear of premature burial led to some very strange quackish practices: medieval doctors would only declare that death had taken place once the body had actually started to rot, a practice that meant perhaps bidding a longer farewell to a deceased relative than most people felt comfortable with, especially as the corpse had to be kept warm in bed until putrefaction set in. Physicians, meanwhile, could run a battery of tests to eliminate the possibility that life flickered, however dimly, in the body of their patient. Invigorating smells, like onion, horseradish and garlic were wafted up the nose. Tobacco smoke could be blown up the anus (one quack even invented a bellows machine to do this), and the skin whipped with nettles. Acrid enemas could be employed, and loud noises and trumpets were blasted in the ears. Vinegar and salt were poured into the mouth, or if none was available, warm urine. Cutting the soles of the feet, dripping hot wax on the head and even the Chauceresque red-hot poker up the bottom were employed. How many people, perhaps hovering at death's door, were ushered over the threshold by these last rites history does not record. After all, what doctor would admit to killing his patient when checking to see if they were dead?

Medicine by Numbers

Throughout the centuries the medical profession has entertained some bizarre notions about the power of numbers, colours and seasons when it comes to treating illness. From Ancient Greece came reams of helpful advice on medical treatments by the calendar. Hippocrates recommended that bleeding and purging take place in spring (in his forty-seventh *Aphorism*). Aetius in the sixth century gave the following instructions for cure of gout, by month:

In September, milk only. October, eat garlic. November, no bathing. December, eat cabbage. January, wine every morning. February, no beets. March, sweets must be mixed with all food and drink. April, avoid horseradish. May, no fish. June, cold water every morning. July, abstinence. August, no mallows.

Anglo-Saxon leechcraft books also had something to say about counting the days until treatment: the first day of March and four days before the end were considered auspicious, for example. This was repeated, with variations, for the whole year. Friday was thought a good day to take medicine, with Good Friday bread being a sovereign cure for most things. The Scots thought illness would always be worst on a Sunday. In Cornwall children with rickets were always bathed on the first Wednesday in May. Things could get more complicated though, as this seventeenth-century example shows: 'Number the dayes from the 26th day of June, to the day when a party first began to fall sick, and divide the number by three; if one remain, he will long be sick; if two, he will die; if none, he will quickly recover.' Apparently this means that only those who fall sick on 4 July will die. Or something like that.

When it came to medicinal colours, red was the physician's colour. Red was regarded as representing heat,

A common medical belief in the Middle Ages was that the body changed every seven years – a spontaneous periodic change in constitution. For example, a man thought choleric might become sanguine. This provided both an easy diagnostic tool for doctors and an effective get-out if they had no idea what was wrong, as any change in health could quite possibly be ascribed to seven-year syndrome.

and white symbolised cold. When people had smallpox, their bed coverings would be red to draw out the pustules to the surface. The son of Edward II was treated in this way at the direction of his physician John of Gaddesden in the fourteenth century. So successful was the treatment that the prince completely recovered, not even scarred by the pox. At the close of the 'eighteenth century, the Emperor Francis, suffering from the same disease, was rolled up in red cloth. It didn't work and he died. Red cords and cloth were important pieces of medical equipment. In the West Indies a strip of scarlet cloth worn around the neck prevents whooping

In such a jungle of misinformation, false trails and downright insanity, it was a thankless task selecting a doctor in the sixteenth century. Happily some advice was available for patients to guide them through the minefield of choosing a healthcare professional. John Halle wrote in 1565 a description, which while not exactly a comprehensive guide, at least provided some hints of what to look out for: 'A surgeon should not be mis-created, deformed, goggle or squint-eye, unhealthy of body, imperfect of mind, not whole in his members, nor boisterous of fingers, or have shaking hands.' A warning we would do well to heed today.

cough. To prevent nosebleeds, a piece of red silk tied around the neck with nine knots is thought helpful. A shrew wrapped in a red rag was a Saxon remedy, but it isn't recorded what it was meant to cure.

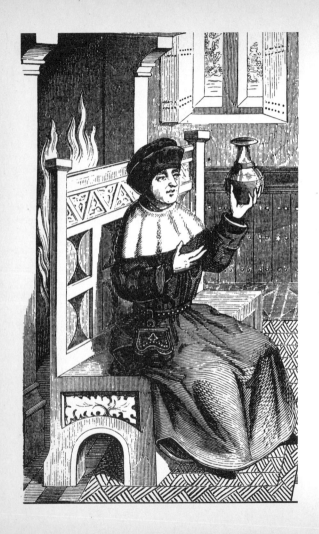

STRANGE FOLK

'Take a young puppy, all one colour, if you can get such a one, and cut him in two pieces through the back alive, and lay one side hot to the grieved place, the inner side I mean.' Thus was gout treated in 1659. Welcome to the world of folk medicine, of bizarre medical treatments, superstition and frogs that could cure blindness.

Away from the world of the fraudulent quack who set out to deliberately defraud and swindle gullible punters, were the thousands of weird cures, which had very little to do with established medicine or making money. These were the folk remedies, handed down over the generations and varying from village to village, often mixed up with old superstitions and magical theories. Some of these strange remedies came from scholars who dabbled in medicine (and were sometimes even proper doctors) and believed that they had perfected infallible medical regimes. John Locke (1632–1704), the great English philosopher, believed, for example, that babies should be bathed in ice-cold water, denied fruit or meat and given only beer to drink. But the majority of these odd cures came from the past, their origins often obscure, but with a discernible taint of ancient magic and ritual. Occasionally

Brotherly love. In the Middle Ages, a certain Robert de Bramwyk had a sister, Denise, who was afflicted with a twisted back and distorted limbs. In an attempt to straighten her out he put her in a cooking pot to soften her up before treading her bones straight.

some remedies, especially herbal ones, were based on sound principles, which must have come from observation of their positive effects on some conditions. Foxglove, for instance, had been used for centuries to treat dropsy (a swelling of the limbs caused by fluid build-up). A derivative is still used today, although more cautiously, to treat the underlying heart problems often responsible for the condition. Another herb, St John's wort, is known as an anti-depressant, and has been used since the fifteenth century. But many folk cures appear to be built on less reasonable foundations.

Tea and Sympathy

The idea of 'sympathetic' cures was well established in folk medicine and even sneaked into the work of some 'men of science'. Sympathetic cures, a kind of medical voodoo, involved diagnosing the cause of a medical complaint and then treating it by focusing attention on a completely separate, but related, object. An example of this concept was the treatment prescribed by the Swiss alchemist Paracelsus (1493–1541) for wounds. He produced a sympathetic ointment, developed no doubt under strict lab conditions, made from 'the moss' of a man's skull, who had been killed or hanged, gathered when Venus was predominant, mixed with red wine and earthworms (other doctors preferred

STRANGE FOLK

'human fat and blood rather than the skull). To use it, one had to find the weapon that had caused the wound to be treated and, it was while still bloody, coat it in ointment. (If the weapon wasn't around, a stick poked in the wound would do.) Repeat four or five times over a course of days. In the meantime the patient should keep the wound covered with a linen rag. By treating the instrument that caused the injury, the wound itself would be 'sympathetically' healed. The story is told of a Captain de Barke, who was treated this way. Injured with shards of glass in his head from a bomb at the siege of Stettin in 1676, he made a full recovery after the shards of glass were extracted and smeared in ointment. Five weeks later he was back in the army – and was promptly killed by a grenade.

A fifth-century tumour cure also relied on sympathy. A root was cut in half and one piece hung around the neck of the patient. The other part was put in the fire; as it shrivelled up, so would the tumour. If the patient was ungrateful, or even refused to pay for the treatment, the doctor could get his revenge by taking the now shrivelled root and reconstituting it in water. As it swelled back up, so the tumour would regrow!

Sympathetic medicine relied heavily on the idea of transference. This meant that the illness could be cured by literally giving it to something else – usually an unfortunate animal. Medieval Frenchmen, for example, would cure tooth-ache by spitting in the mouth of a frog. In seventeenth-century Ireland, a live trout, placed in the mouth of a child with whooping cough, then thrown back into the river, would carry off the disease. If trout was off the menu, then a frog was an acceptable substitute. If both trout and frogs were hard to come by, a simple mug of water, taken against the current, would suffice. The child was to drink one mouthful then throw

'Warty eruptions', claimed the tenth-century monks of Glastonbury Abbey, could be treated by a virgin hanging seven wafers around the neck. By the late Middle Ages this advice had changed and it was agreed by the cognoscenti that a piece of stolen beef rubbed on the warts and then buried in 'filth' would ensure they went away. Countryside cures espoused suitably rustic wart remedies – spiking snails and watching them dry was thought to be a good way to banish them, as was tying a horse's hair around the warty bump. Throwing a piece of knotted string, one knot for each wart, in an outside privy would also apparently get rid of them.

the rest away, and repeat this for three consecutive mornings before the break of dawn.

Jamaican folk medicine recommended that a live, large, hairless black dog stretched out over the body of a feverish patient would suck the illness into itself, while in Ancient Greece it was enough to be licked by one of the dogs of the temple of Ascelpius (the Greek god of healing) to get rid of ill-health.

Some cures could be quite elaborate, as this seventeenth-century remedy for fever from Sir Kenelm Digby, medical dilettante and diplomat, demonstrates: 'Pare the patient's nails; put the parings in a little bag, and hang the bag around

In 1877 a report appeared in a newspaper about a Kentucky farmer who possessed a mad-stone, sold to him by an Italian. When a person was bitten by a mad dog, they were brought to the house and the mad-stone rubbed on the bite. After this it was soaked in warm milk. In twenty-three years it cured fifty-nine people.

One common whooping cough cure was to take the hair from the head of the ill person, put it into a sandwich and feed it to a dog. It was believed that as the dog choked on the hair and tried to cough it up, it would somehow assume the disease from the child.

the neck of a live eel, and place him in a tub of water. The eel will die, the patient will recover.' Unlikely as it was that anyone suffering from fever and ague could be bothered to go fishing for eels in the first place, the question of whether eels actually have necks and if they do where they begin and end, vital to this cure, is also sadly left unanswered.

It wasn't just the Europeans who were transferring all their illnesses to any passing creatures. Victorian anthropologists diligently recorded bizarre local customs from all over the Empire. Hindus, they noted, had very elaborate rituals for getting rid of jaundice, which involved banishing the condition's yellow colour to the places it properly belonged – like parrots, thrushes and the sun. Plutarch (45–125 AD) noted that if jaundiced people stared at a stone-curlew, and the bird stared back at them, 'it draws out and receives the malady, which issues, like a stream, through the eyesight'. Merchants who sold the birds at market soon became wise to this, and to stop jaundiced people getting a free cure, kept the cages with the stone-curlews in them covered with a cloth at all times.

Preposterous Prophylactics

Prevention, of course, is better than cure, and folk medicine embraced this doctrine most heartily. All sorts of weird and wonderful substances and rituals were used to ward off

QUACK MAGIC

An old Sussex remedy advised that to prevent the ague a necklace made from the wooden chips of a gallows would make an effective prophylactic, although if such wooden jewellery was felt to be a fashion faux pas, a man's woollen sock, filled with earthworms, could be worn instead.

disease. Some of them involved a sort of reverse transference, where some mysterious power ascribed to an object or animal could be acquired and used to prevent illness (and in some cases cure it as well). This was obviously the case of the medieval folk who fancied setting themselves up as eye specialists – they were advised to procure a frog. By licking its eyes, any subsequent human eyes they licked would be instantly cured. Folklore also claimed that having pierced ears (golden rings only) stopped eye disease developing. Other preventative measures were based purely on superstition, like the Victorian woman from Manchester who requested a pinch of clay from the grave of a priest to ward off epilepsy in her children.

Creosote and tar were for a long time considered good for opening up the lungs, a sort of 'changing the air', which would help strengthen the chest and prevent infection. Not content with packing pasty urban waifs off to the seaside for a healthy blast of ozone and sea bathing, mothers would march their children down to the local gasworks to inhale deep draughts of the fumes in the first half of the twentieth century. The tar-scented air around road-surfacing works was also valued as a cheap medicine for children with, or in danger of getting, whooping cough, who would stand by the hot vats of bubbling bitumen and breathe in the pungent vapours. Pieces of stray tar could be chewed or sucked. If

OZONE PAPER

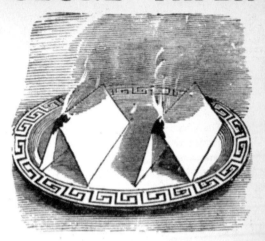

Magic rings, not just the preserve of hobbits and elves, played a significant part in medicine, folk and mainstream. The physician and alchemist Paracelsus had a medical ring forged, which he claimed cured not only cramp but palsy, epilepsy and apoplexy. Rings made from the hinges of coffins were supposed to help cramp according to sixteenth-century medical lore and Henry VIII was believed to own one. In 1794 *Gentleman's* magazine carried an article which instructed that a silver ring made from five sixpences, collected from five different bachelors and conveyed by the hand of a bachelor to a smith who was a bachelor, would cure fits!

a piece of tarred rope could be found, all the better, as carrying this around this provided a handy pocket-sized preventative.

Cramp could be prevented by putting a piece of potato or brimstone under the mattress. Alternatively a rusty sword hung on the wall by the bed would ensure a cramp-free night and provide an attractive decorative feature too. Scottish folk medicine decreed that a mole's paw or sheep's tooth carried around would prevent toothache.

Animal magic

Medicine and animals go back a long way. After all, the Hippocratic emblem of medicine and doctors is a snake curled around a staff (the symbol of Ascelpius). Man has always used animals in medicine, both mainstream and unorthodox. Ancient shamans used animal parts in their potions, and even today medical research and testing is often carried out on animals, with animal parts being used in modern medicines and surgical techniques.

STRANGE FOLK

One particularly bizarre sixteenth-century remedy for wounds was a 'mysterious compound' – *oleum catellorum* – live cats boiled in olive oil.

In studying the use of animals in historical medicine, it soon becomes obvious that all creatures weren't created equal in the eyes of the practitioners. Squirrels, for example, hardly get a mention, but the unlucky hare was a firm favourite for all sorts of remedies.

The Saxons were particularly keen on it, using different parts of its body for a variety of treatments: its brain, stewed in wine, promoted sleep; the lungs could be removed and bound over sore eyes; carrying around its ankle bone warded off cramp. The Chinese believed that the hare sat under a special tree by the light of the moon, manufacturing the drugs required for immortality, making it a must-have pet for any aspiring quack. The pastern bone of a hare, according to fourth-century folklore, was good for infant colic if it a) was found in the dung of a wolf; b) had had no contact with the ground; and c) hadn't been touched by a woman.

Dogs didn't fare much better. The right foot shank of a dead black dog (black animals are valued highly in the weird medicine sector) hung jauntily over the arm was supposed to banish fever, whereas the head of a mad dog pounded and

A sixth-century cure for cataracts urged the patient to catch a fox. While it was still alive, its tongue was to be torn out. The fox could then be released (if still alive), but the tongue should be kept on the sufferer's person wrapped in a red rag.

mixed with wine cured jaundice, alternatively burnt and the ashes put on a tumour was reputed to cure cancer. The eighteenth-century evangelist John Wesley recommended holding a live puppy on the stomach to relieve constipation. European clinical practice said that if a person was bitten by a mad dog, then on no account could it be left to run away. Instead it had to be caught and its liver torn out and pressed to the wound to ensure healing, and the heart cut out and baked, before being ground up and made into an infusion to drink. In 1866 a woman testified at an inquest that her child had contracted hydrophobia after being bitten by a rabid dog. Having requested that the body of the dog, which had been drowned by townspeople nine days previously, be dredged up, she then cut out its liver and fed it to her child, but unfortunately this wasn't successful. A cake baked with the heart of a white dog was said to aid people who suffered from fits and convulsions.

Horses didn't escape the butchery either. Mongolians would cure foot complaints by thrusting their feet into the warm entrails of a freshly killed nag, and the stuff inside a horse's hoof, dissolved, was used in medieval Kent as a remedy for ague. However, the horse was an expensive animal, and so generally they were left alive, with just bits

The first successful blood transfusion was carried out in 1665 by Richard Lower, when he successfully moved blood between two dogs. Emboldened by his success he overreached somewhat and next attempted an inter-species transfusion, this time from a lamb to a man. Alas, he discovered that ovine and human blood are not interchangeable, and both guinea-pigs died.

In the late sixteenth century, a man named Peter Lelen was suddenly taken ill with weakness and pain 'in his sydes'. Different medicines were administered, but all seemed to have no effect. In desperation the physician decided to try an experimental new concoction – horse dung and beer. As soon as the patient tasted it, a violent reaction was noted; 'it made all the blood in his veins boil, and put all his humours into such a general fermentation that he seemed to be in a boiling kettle'. Miraculously, he was cured, although doctors noticed that the drug had left some side effects, namely that afterwards Peter 'coveted strong ale mightily'.

snipped off for medical essentials – such as swallowing horsehair for worms.

Old-fashioned physicians, it seems, would kill just about anything when it came to devising remedies. Pigeons had numerous medical uses, which Samuel Pepys noticed when he went to visit the sickly Catherine, wife of Charles II, in 1663. He noted how unwell she looked and remarked that pigeons had been set at her feet as an indication of how dangerously ill she was. His diary tells of another visit a few years later to see a dying friend whose 'breath rattled in his throat, and they did lay pigeons at his feet, and all despair of him'. This bizarre medical practice came from the idea that pigeons were connected with death, and a person could not take leave of life if they were lying on pigeon feathers. The French favoured the pigeon not just for the pot, but for a whole range of therapeutic uses: they could, for instance, be clapped to the heads of mad people, and their blood dripped warm on to the flanks for relief of pleurisy. The blood from the wings of the young birds was thought very good for the eyes.

Skinned mice were swallowed by the Ancient Egyptians as a medicine of last resort. Remains of mice have been found in the alimentary canals of child skeletons, indicating that they had died before being able to fully digest the medicinal rodent. In seventeenth-century Lincolnshire, fried mice were fed to children with whooping cough.

Handy Home Cures

'Every man his own doctor,' declared one eighteenth-century home remedy compendium. Sadly, in the modern world where medicine rests in the hands of the pro-fessionals, much of this folklore is forgotten and people will rush to their doctor for the slightest complaint. Science and the information age have conspired to make us all hypochondriacs, alert to every little twinge and worried that

Part of the reasoning behind the foul substances used in some cures came down to the simple belief that one evil would drive out another. The more horrid they were, the more memorable the cure. Thus pioneer Americans in the Midwest would cheerfully imbibe nanny tea – made from sheep's dung – in cases of measles. Fits in babies were treated with twenty to forty grains from the scrapings of pewter spoons. Bear's gall in rum was an accepted cure of the time for hysterical people, who were also advised to supplement their diet with gold filings. Diarrhoea called for the 'yard or pizzle' (penis) of a buck, dried, powdered, infused in raw spirit and sipped until the going went from soft to firm. Bad breath could be masked with an early morning gargle of urine – your own, of course.

it signals some life-threatening illness. Knowledge is in an inverse relationship with medicine; rather than empowering us, it seems the more we find out about illness and disease, the less able we are to deal with it ourselves. In an attempt to restore the balance a little, here are a few remedies for some of the everyday (and a few not so common) complaints you may suffer.

Asthma
An old Arabic cure recommends taking dried and powdered fox lung with figs. The Romans preferred owl's blood for this condition.

Common Cold
Rather than just blowing a stuffy hooter, why not try the old folk idea of stuffing orange peel up each nostril? If troubled by a sore throat, then perhaps this old country cure is worth a stab: tie a stocking, the dirtier the better, round the neck before going to bed. If a stocking isn't available then a dirty sock will suffice, but remember that the heel must be over the larynx if the cure is to work. If, for some reason, neither stocking or sock are available, then a thick piece of toast soaked in vinegar can be bound on with a handkerchief.

Chest Complaints
An old English remedy for a bad chest is to take the sufferer to a field of cows early in the morning. When a cow arises from its night's sleep, the ill person immediately should lie down in the warm space just vacated, and inhale the lingering bovine aroma deeply. Good health will soon be restored. Alternatively, simply inhaling the breath of cattle will relieve some chest complaints. Of course, prevention is better than

cure and pigs can be just as effective as cows. Bronchial trouble can be warded off by wearing a piece of bacon strapped to the ribcage. Or a cunning vest of goose fat and brown paper may be fashioned, to be sported at all times 'wearable until the smell becomes unbearable'. To be extra certain of avoiding chest complaints, greasing the soles of the feet is an additional precaution, although hazardous when walking on smooth surfaces or downhill.

Chills, Fever and Ague

Fever can be cured by pills, specifically the little woodlice that roll into balls when touched, hence their name 'pill-bugs'. If this cure doesn't appeal, then like the old lady in the nursery rhyme, a live spider should be taken. For squeamish types who may not be able to stomach an active arachnid in their gullet, an alternative is placing the spider in a bag round the neck. Parson James Woodforde (1740–1803) took a more robust attitude towards the feverish. In his diary he describes

Fever can, of course, be more serious than just a common cold. A report from 1883 tells of a Turkish upholsterer who was struck down by typhoid. Suffering a terrible fever, he developed a raging thirst. In his delirium he wandered into a kitchen where he tried to quench it by drinking the vinegar from a bucket of pickled cabbage. Miraculously he somehow recovered from the disease. Doctors immediately pronounced that pickled cabbage juice was a cure for typhoid, a position they soon had to revise when a number of patients who had the same illness inconveniently died despite taking this new remedy. Cabbage juice, backtracked the medical men, did cure typhoid, but only in upholsterers.

the cure he inflicted on a suffering relative who came to visit: 'I gave him a dram of gin at the beginning of the fit and pushed him headlong into one of my ponds, then ordered him to bed immediately.' What a host. People in eighteenth-century Sussex were likely to be recommended seven sage leaves each morning of a seven-day fast.

Whooping Cough

Wandering from one county in England to the next reveals different historical ways of curing this now rare disease. Seemingly, each region was in competition with the others to be crowned winner in a 'strangest local remedy' contest. In Norfolk, for instance, a spider was prescribed, tied up in a muslin cloth and hung over the mantelpiece. In Yorkshire, locals favoured a savoury broth made from owls and fed to an afflicted child, whereas Suffolk folk would take boys and girls to be dipped head first in a hole freshly cut in a meadow. West Country types would bake the cake from hell – made from barley and child's urine, a medicine likely to need more than a spoonful of sugar to help it down. For someone who couldn't be bothered to research the best local remedies, there were national guidelines. In England the consensus was that riding a bear would cure whooping cough, while those north of the border favoured following the instructions of any man who passed by on a piebald horse. This cure for 'hooping cough' comes from the sister-in-law of Jane Austen, Martha Lloyd: 'Cut off the hair from the top of the head as large as a crown piece. Take a piece of brown paper of the same size: dip it in rectified oyl of amber, and apply it to the part for nine mornings, dipping the paper fresh each morning. If the cough is not removed, try it again after three or four days.'

Broken Bones

Comfrey tea is advised by most folk remedies as a way of getting broken bones to knit. Alternatively, the powdered dust of dog's skull was recommended in one Victorian anthology of rural medicine. In the sixteenth century, sticks used to be thrust between the breaks of bones to actually stop them knitting, the painful consequences considered necessary evidence that healing was under way.

Cuts and Wounds

A stone, heated and dropped in a bucket of water, which is then used to wash, will help heal wounds and bruises. Tobacco, mouldy bread, mashed earthworms in calf's dung and toasted cheese are all recommended folk cures for treating minor cuts and grazes. Medieval medical practice believed wholeheartedly in not letting wounds heal up; instead the skin was doused in acids and the flaps of a wound held apart with leaden tubes and 'tents'. The skin would be cut away and plugged so it could not heal, and wounds would be dilated with huge forceps to tear the flesh apart and achieve the painful suppuration considered vital for healing.

Spider's webs were renowned for their excellent wound-stopping properties. French soldiers used to carry spider's webs in their packs for this purpose, and Robert Burton in his 1621 *Anatomy of Melancholy* tells of how his scepticism of this old cure was overcome when he watched his mother dress a wound with spiders' web – with instant effects.

Headaches

Onions, cut and rubbed on the temples, are claimed to relieve headaches. A piece from a hangman's rope, worn as a

A historical snippet, which doesn't demonstrate the intellectual capacities of students in the best light, tells of a man who, in the days of Queen Victoria, sat on the steps of King's College chapel in Cambridge and sold snake skins, which could be bound round the head as a cure for headache, no doubt aimed at the market of academics who had been too long at their books. Or in the pub.

headband can also see off a throbbing skull. The Greeks and Romans both used electric eels and fish to give shocks to the head, believing this would help. A fourth-century cure recommended swallowing the stones found in the stomachs of small birds, and eighteenth-century medicine books recommend a poultice of raw potato as an analgesic. For headaches caused by physical damage this diagnostic technique from fifteenth-century Italy was inspired by violinmakers. Patients would clench a string between their teeth, which the surgeon would pull taut and pluck. If a clear tone was heard, then the skull was deemed to be intact; a dull twanging signalled a fracture.

Opium poppies are effective in curing a headache. Less strong then their Far Eastern counterparts, they grow in the English countryside and were at one time sold at Ely market. The local Fenmen were castigated as being 'small, slothful and dull-witted', possibly as a result of their poppy habit.

Sight and Sound

For sore eyes and incipient blindness, take a leaf from the book of the ancients. Egyptian doctors favoured the gall bladder of a pig for eye infections – cut in half and left on the face overnight then dried, powdered and rubbed into the eyeball. Severe cases called for the mixing of the eyes of the unfortunate pig

Strangely omitted from modern textbooks on ocular treatments, spitting has a long and noble history as a cure for eye disease. The Emperor Vespasian (AD 9–79) cured a blind man by spitting in his eyes, and Captain James Cook tried the same trick on a local when he landed in America. An old folk cure calls for the spittle of a fasting peasant.

with honey, and placing them overnight in the ear of the patient. Ingrowing eyelashes were coated with a salve of bat's and lizard's blood. According to folk rumour, having pierced ears helps stave off eye problems, but if troubled by a stye then rubbing it with the golden wedding ring of your spouse can help, or for the unmarried, applying blood drawn from the tail of a black cat.

Human excrement, dried and powdered, has long been used as a remedy for eye problems. Unsuccessfully. A more pleasant remedy is the eighteenth-century idea of drinking a large draught of beer every morning.

For ear complaints a clove of garlic, dipped in honey and left overnight in the ear would address minor problems, claimed one rustic cure. Black wool was an alternative ear-stuffing, as was the juice from snails (which was something of a cure-all) and a cockroach dipped in oil. For really persistent ear troubles nothing could beat ant eggs, steeped in onion juice and packed deep in the ear canal.

An old English recipe for an earache cure. Take one hedgehog. Kill it. Pluck or shave off its spines and slowly heat the bald carcass over a fire until it begins to drip. Catch this 'oil' and pour it into the troubled ear for a complete cure.

Toothache and Mouth Problems

Snake skins, soaked in vinegar and chewed, were considered a toothache cure in seventeenth-century Wales. Henbane (incidentally, used by Dr Crippen to murder his wife), thrown on the fire and the vapour inhaled, could also relieve the pain. Of course, regular brushing could help prevent tooth troubles, and Hippocrates, the father of medicine, had his own special toothpaste made from cooked-up mice and hare's head. The hand of a dead man or the tooth of a horse were both believed to remove dental discomfort.

Stuttering was thought to be cured by having the end of the tongue snipped off – recommended by eighteenth-century German doctors. Children were often taken to the doctor to have the 'bridle' – the soft part underneath – of their tongue cut. This operation was popular for any sort of speech impediment, and was carried out far more than was really necessary for the very occasional cases that warranted this treatment. One Victorian doctor in Manchester took to sending away the parents who brought young girls to him for this procedure. A woman who couldn't talk, he grandly asserted, would be desired by men when it came to finding a husband later on.

Baby Care

Much folkish wisdom surrounds raising babies. After all, it was widely believed that the Roman Emperor Caligula was bloodthirsty because his wet-nurse had daubed blood on her nipples before suckling him. Wet-nurses had an important role in the life of children in their care. Menstruating women were not permitted to be wet-nurses in the seventeenth century, and doctors decreed that 'sluttish' wet-nurses and midwives caused rickets. Women who had a squint, kidney

The Church controlled the licensing of midwives in England, as the Royal College of Physicians would have nothing to do with them. Licences bound midwives, amongst other things, not to use sorcery or incantations and not to pull the heads off any babies. Decorum was paramount in the delivery room, and many women refused men entry. Peter Willoughby, a seventeenth-century doctor from Derby, would creep unseen into the delivery room on his hands and knees.

stones and bad breath were well advised to choose another career, as well as those with irregular opinions or religious beliefs. Wet-nurses were understood to transfer all their ideas and feelings to the suckling child. Samuel Johnson blamed his wet-nurse for his bad eyesight.

To promote easier birth, women should be strapped to a board, which was then banged on the ground to promote delivery. Nicholas Culpeper recommended women labour in a darkened room because 'labour weakens her eyes exceedingly by a harmony between the womb and them'.

A TURN FOR THE WORSE

Consumption, 'the white plague', has also been called the 'Captain of Death'. Even today someone will die of the disease every fifteen seconds, and throughout history it has claimed countless lives. Victims of the disease have been discovered in excavations as far back as Ancient Egypt, and England in 1780 lost 1.25 per cent of its entire population to the disease. In the early nineteenth century it was estimated that at least a quarter of Europe had the disease, and today perhaps up to one-third of the world's inhabitants is infected

 Tuberculosis or consumption is spread by the bacteria *mycobacterium tuberculosis*. TB usually occurs as pneumonia, but it can also appear in the brain, back, knee, lymph nodes, or other organs and bones. Highly infectious, it is spread by breathing infected air, usually in close proximity to a coughing sufferer. Common symptoms include a severe cough, fevers, night sweats, and unexplained weight loss.

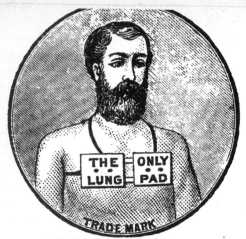

ABSOLUTELY CURES
Consumption, Asthma, Bronchitis, and all diseases of the Throat, Lungs and Chest.

A POSITIVE, EFFECTUAL and RADICAL CURE.

WRITE FOR TESTIMONIALS.

Sold by Druggists, or sent on receipt of price, $2.00.

THE ONLY LUNG PAD CO.,
DETROIT, MICH.

Other Roman cures for TB included bathing in human urine, drinking elephant's blood and eating wolves livers.

with the germ that causes tuberculosis, according to the World Health Organisation.

Hippocrates recognised TB as a specific disease, and Ancient Greek physicians noted the consumptive type – pale, thin and narrow-chested – an observation borne out in modern studies, which have demonstrated that fat people may be less susceptible to consumption. Treatment revolved around building up the strength of the patient – preparations like 'the lard of a thin sow, the flesh of an ass and the ashes of a pig's tongue' were all prescribed with a view to making the patient hardy and thick-skinned. These ideas were further developed by the Romans, who recommended a warm climate, sea voyages and plenty of milk to strengthen the patient, ideas that held sway from the second century BC until the twentieth century AD.

Most families would have some experience of consumption, and it was no respecter of rank or talent. St Francis of Assisi, Keats, Chopin, Eleanor Roosevelt, assorted Brontës and many others succumbed to the disease. Although infectious, it didn't always affect people in the same way. Keats, famously, was dead within eleven months of contracting the disease, whereas his fellow writer Robert Louis Stevenson lasted for decades before expiring.

Off to the Sanatorium

Such a widespread disease, and one which could potentially go on for so long before the patient recovered or died, meant that there was plenty of opportunity for medical experimentation. Mainstream medicine relied on the old ideas of a change in climate, setting off to sea and the consumption of milk in heroic quantities. A gut-busting sixteen glasses a day with twelve eggs wasn't unusual in some sanatoriums. Of course, it didn't help that for years, doctors had been certain that consumption was hereditary and not spread by infection. Northern Europeans were puzzled when travelling to Italy and Spain, where, by the early eighteenth century, controls had been established on the movements of tubercular people to limit infections. Surely this was unnecessary for an hereditary disease? The usual bleedings and purges were also given to consumptive patients, no doubt dangerously weakening them and in some cases hastening their demise. Thomas Sydenham, the seventeenth-century doctor who was called 'the English Hippocrates', recommended horseback riding as a cure for consumption. His exalted position in the medical firmament at the time meant that his contemporaries unquestioningly adopted his ideas. For years all consumptives were prescribed a canter on horseback for their complaint, and even Keats, at death's door in 1820, was hoisted aboard for a restorative trot.

Grandmother's Cures

With consumption so prevalent, people were susceptible to new cures that offered some hope. Perhaps like no other single disease, quackish and bizarre remedies have gathered round consumption like microbes on sputum.

One of the strangest remedies for tuberculosis of the lymph glands of the neck – scrofula – was the belief that it could be cured by the touch of a royal hand, a power claimed by both British and French monarchs. Only a touch from the monarch would do though; lesser royals just didn't have the same powers, and the disease became known as 'the King's evil'. Prominent royal touchers were Edward the Confessor, who brought the practice to England, and Louis XIV of France, who was said to have touched over 2,000 diseased subjects. Most diligent was perhaps Charles II, who processed 92,000 people under the royal hand between 1662 and 1682. One famous 'touchee' was Samuel Johnson, who was taken by his mother in 1712 to London to be healed by Queen Anne, the last British monarch to still regularly carry out the practice. He received the royal touch, and also a 'touch piece', a gold token given by the court to everyone who was touched, and was thought to have some inherent curative powers of its own. Obviously being touched came with no sort of guarantee of cure, as Dr Johnson was to discover in later life when he underwent draining surgery on his infected lymph glands.

Other methods of cure were available for those who couldn't get close to the sovereign. People who moved in the wrong circles had to make do with more homespun remedies.

The ancient view of a change in the climate to cure consumption caused some division in the medical world. Following the Greeks, some physicians recommended a warm and balmy atmosphere – Robert Louis Stephenson, for example, headed south for the Pacific Islands. But other physicians recommended cold air, alpine if possible, to chill and cool the lungs. This led to the fashion in the early twentieth century for open-air schools for consumptive children.

QUACK MAGIC

An old English consumption cure. Take one good cock. Tear it apart while it is still alive and flatten the pieces with a goodly club. Put the pieces in a pot, and place this pot inside a bigger pot. Add herbs, dates, gold and a handful of pearls. Consume and be cured.

One advised tying the leaves of a particular plant to the leg of a cock or a dog with string. The animal was then supposed to pull the plant from the ground as it wandered off; for the person to uproot it would be fatal, of course. Once the plant was out, the juice had to be squeezed from the leaves and drunk every Wednesday morning, and the discarded plant burnt. Woodbines were required in an old Scottish cure, although not for smoking; passing a consumptive through a woodbine wreath would make them well. Swallowing slugs could apparently work wonders.

Cows played a big part in consumption cures. In Ancient Greece, milk and other dairy products were thought soothing and good for increasing a patient's strength. Butter made from the milk of cows that grazed in churchyards was especially helpful, as was their milk. The air in a cow barn was good for the consumptive soul, and in 1820s America, TB patients were placed in rooms built just above cattle stalls as a form of treatment. However, some experts suggest that bovine tuberculosis could have provided the source of infection for early TB sufferers.

A list of consumption cures from an 1818 American pioneer medicine book includes: cow heels with ginger; gruel and water; buttermilk and white bread; and sucking on the breasts of a healthy woman.

A TURN FOR THE WORSE

The Expert Quack

John St John Long was perhaps one of the most famous quacks of the Victorian era. A charming and handsome Irishman, he made his name as a specialist for the consumptive. He had no shortage of patients. TB was rife in the nineteenth century and highly infectious; just a droplet of spit was enough to spread the disease.

Long had developed a special 'medicine' that was to be rubbed on to the patient. If nothing happened, then the patient was well. But if there was a skin reaction, from redness through to blistering, then the patient was obviously ill; the change in their skin was a sign of the disease being 'extracted'. If the patient did not recover quickly then more rubbing with the ointment was required. In particularly bad cases, special inhalations could also be prescribed from a device Long had set up in his surgery. When the disease was under control the skin was allowed to heal under the daily application of a few cabbage leaves.

Long soon became a rich man. His Harley Street practice was crowded with patients, and the cream of society came to

 Having consumption wasn't all bad news. For a while in the nineteenth century the 'consumptive look' – pale and interesting – was highly fashionable and became a romanticised ideal. William Morris painted a peaky-looking Guinevere, and opera presented beautiful and consumption-stricken characters such as Violetta in *La Traviata*. Perhaps most famously, Lord Byron flirted with the idea of death by consumption, not least so he could impress the ladies with his new look while on his deathbed.

Quack consumption cures may have flourished because of the apparently heightened response of TB sufferers to placebo medicine. A French physician, Dr Mathieu, demonstrated this when he carried out trials; he told TB sufferers under his care that a new consumption remedy had been discovered – 'Antiphymose'. This was just a salt solution, but to the patients he gave it to the effect was noticeable; their appetite improved, coughs and night sweats diminished, and the need to hawk up spit was curbed.

seek his opinion. Critical of established medical practitioners, Long soon accumulated a number of enemies, irritated by his success and his outspoken attacks. Most doctors, he said, were greedy fools who would prolong a patient's suffering in order to inflate their bills. They purchased their qualifications with no study, prescribed dangerous drugs like mercury, and relied on painful and outdated treatments such as bleeding and purging. Long, on the other hand, made great virtue of the fact that his treatments were gentle and had no unpleasant effects. However, this wasn't quite true, and his enemies soon got their chance to attack him when his rubbing cure was shown to be rather harsher than he claimed. An Irish patient, Miss Cashin, had come to England specifically to see Long about her consumption. He attended her and prescribed his usual treatment, rubbing his patent cure over her back. However, it soon became very inflamed and refused to heal; the girl refused any further treatment and grew dangerously unwell. The most prominent physician in London was called, the Queen's own surgeon, but with no success and Miss Cashin died the next day.

Long's enemies celebrated and he was soon taken to court on a manslaughter charge. But he was not alone; many of his famous clientele turned up to support him. Despite having their celebrity weight behind him – including one eminent man who sat next to the judge throughout the trial chatting to him, no doubt about what an excellent cove Long was – the jury found him guilty and he was fined £250. Insolently Long pulled the money from his pocket in the dock and paid his fine then and there, walking away from court a free man. The post-mortem was inconclusive and Long himself claimed that the young woman had died through an over-fondness for ripe fruit, a diagnosis that seemed to wash with his patients as his practice was undiminished by this escapade. His enemies must have gnashed their teeth in frustration, but they were soon to get another chance to have a crack at John St John Long. Almost his next patient after the trial was a Mrs Lloyd who suffered from a throat complaint of uncertain origin. Her lungs, however, were free from consumption. Nonetheless, Dr Long prescribed inhalations and rubbing of her throat and chest. As soon as he had completed this, a violent reaction occurred; redness and blistering with discharge spread across the whole area. Cabbage leaves were hastily applied and Long advised her to continue with the rubbing treatment. Mrs Lloyd, though, couldn't bear any more of his ministrations 'and declined to see him any more'. Within a month of her first treatment she was dead, with a huge ulcer stretching 'from the armpits across the chest in one direction and from the collar bones to under the nipples in the other'.

It was back to the Old Bailey for Long, but again he was acquitted. This time, though, business was damaged, with patients understandably worried by a doctor whose frequent court appearances did little for their confidence. His famous friends rallied round, signing a petition protesting the

It was thought beneficial in the eighteenth century to have asthma. People who did were believed to be immune from TB.

excellence of his medicine, claiming that they all had used his rubbing lotion with no ill effects. Long died, still a very wealthy man, in 1834 at the young age of thirty-six. Ironically, he died of consumption, doubtless contracted from one of his patients.

Of course, if you couldn't afford the doctor, and were fed up with folk remedies, there were still lots of cures to try. The quacks who sold the thousands of different consumption cures were also selling 'science' – potions and pills concocted specifically for the relief of consumption. With sea journeys, mountain air, sanatoriums and even a visit to a quack like Long out of the reach of the coughing masses, many turned to the wonder cures, which promised so much. A bewildering number of medicines were available, on both sides of the Atlantic. One such was peddled by Newcastle merchant George Handyside, who was making his fortune on the back of his 1858 'Cure for Consumption', one of a stable of medicines marketed by the Geordie shoemaker, builder, advertising executive and quack medicine entrepreneur. His 'Blood Purifier' and 'Blood Food' were also popular, but the consumption medicine was the jewel in the crown. Each bottle depicted sickly people queuing to cross a bridge (the consumption cure), upon the other side of which the newly restored strode off, in the pink of health.

Other great British products were also available. Hagues Kure-a-Kof, Bronkura, Lowe's Manchester Cough Cure (proof absolute that it was grim up north) and Liqufruta Cough Cure were just a few of the medicines around. For

Liqufruta is still available from chemists today, although in a different incarnation. Nowadays its ingredients are clearly listed, with no unidentified sticky matter floating within.

the most part they contained water flavoured with a few herbs and bits and pieces. Some would contain opium, useful as a cough suppressant, but usually such medicines would flaunt their narcotic content openly and be sold on this benefit separately as a 'soothing' medicine. In the case of Liqufruta, when analysed by a Victorian chemist, its contents revealed that it was a mixture of onion, water, sugar and an unidentifiable 'mucilaginous matter', which begs the question of whether some sufferer had coughed *into* the bottle by mistake.

In the US it was a similar picture. One of the most famous consumption cures available was Dr Kilmer's Indian Cough Cure and Consumption Oil, which claimed to 'definitely and positively' cure consumption. The Kilmer brothers, Jonas and 'Prof' S. Andral Kilmer (claiming, fraudulently of course, a medical degree), concocted their oil, and sold such volumes of product that they were able to open a bottling plant in Binghampton, New York, turning out thousands of gallons of the stuff. In 1892 the Prof left the company to set up his 'Cancertorium', a venture purporting to cure all types of cancer for those rich enough to buy a place there. Nonetheless the company still continued to turn out its popular oil for vast profit until new legislation in 1906 forced it to disclose the ingredients on the labels. Like many of the cures of the day, the Kilmers had included more than a dash of alcohol in their 'medicine', and once people could see what was actually in it, sales soon declined. Nonetheless, the

QUACK MAGIC

Some of the cures available were highly dangerous. Lung Germine was a consumption cure which offered 'proof that will convince any judge or jury on earth' of its powers. It was certainly powerful, made of a lethal mixture of sulphuric acid and alcohol.

Kilmer name was still powerful enough to shift enough medicine to keep the company afloat for a while. It is still possible to buy bottles of Dr Kilmer's Swamp Oil today, although it is sold just as a tonic drink and seems to have lost its consumption-curing powers.

Other fraudsters also made TB-curing hay. One with an interesting past was Orlando Edgar Miller, an American quack who at the end of the nineteenth century dabbled in various cures before settling on consumption as his speciality. Inconveniently detained in prison halfway through his career for selling a patent rupture cure, upon release he set up a business selling 'medicated sand' as a cure for dyspepsia. He also established a society, St Luke's, which he claimed to have philanthropic and religious motives and which was dedicated to the cure of those addicted to morphine, tobacco and strong liquor. Whatever this philanthropy was, it paid well and he soon had a large sanatorium, which was doing good business until it unfortunately burned down, taking thirteen inmates with it. Undeterred he set up a new institute, known grandly as Ruskin University, where patients could come for 'every known process of healing'. This venture, though, was sadly not a success after the mud bath treatments advertised were in fact discovered to be nothing more than a splash through the local swamp. Orlando E. was fined and told to leave town, but as one establishment closed, another soon mushroomed up. This next venture was 'The International Institute for the Treatment of Tuberculosis', and was the Xanadu of his quackish foundations. The treatment offered was unique, claimed Miller, 'a combination of vegetable substances, which, administered hypodermatically, produces three effects on the system, viz: Sleep, Relaxation, Elimination'. Advertisements took the form of specially concocted 'case reports', which told of the treatment's marvellous results. This was slightly undermined in 1908 when one special 'case report' on a Raymond Forsyth was published, which claimed he was well on the road to recovery from TB after taking the cure. Bizarrely, a local newspaper simultaneously carried an obituary for poor Raymond after he had died following, 'an extended illness covering two years'. Alarmed, the authorities investigated Miller's Institute, in particular his claims that he enjoyed an 80 per cent success rate in curing consumption. Alas, statistical analysis wasn't his strength; contrary to his claims, investigators found that of fifty-one people who had been treated by Miller for the illness, thirty-six were dead and three were in the final stages of the disease. Of the remaining twelve no further trace of them could be found, a circumstance

Other nineteenth-century cures for TB included Prof Hoff's, Nature's Creation, Tuberculoids, Bromin-Iodin, Oxidaze and Hydrocine. All continued to be sold in the first part of the twentieth century, until advances in real medicine started to make inroads on the disease, based on the discovery of the responsible TB germ. However, the threat of the disease hasn't gone away, even if the quacks have. AIDS has ensured that TB is once again on the increase. By 2005 an estimated 12 million new cases of TB will have emerged.

that didn't bode well. Disgraced, Miller disappeared from view, to London, in fact, from where reports came that he had opened a sanatorium!

Cancer Quacks

Old quacks would think nothing of adding cancer to the list of diseases their patent medicines could claim to banish. Tonics, salves, cordials and balms had outrageous claims made about their healing powers, and were, of course, completely ineffective. The logic was the more illnesses your medicine could cure, the more people would buy it.

However, some unscrupulous charlatans went a step further, and set themselves up as cancer specialists, with an arsenal of 'scientific' products at their disposal. At best ineffective, and at worst positively lethal, quack cancer remedies often hastened the end of the patients using them.

Rupert Wells (or Dennis Dupuis to give him his real name), operating in the US around 1907, claimed he had developed a secret remedy for cancer. His credentials sounded impressive; he was Chair of Radiotherapy at the prestigious Postgraduate College of Electrotherapeutics of St Louis. However, for such an august faculty it had a surprisingly low membership. Just one, in fact; 'Dr' Wells himself. The whole establishment and its mythical chair were a fiction he invented to provide good advertising copy. This was vital, as

 According to folk medicine, cancer could be cured by taking the scrapings from a brass kettle, mixing them with mutton fat and plastering the paste over the affected area.

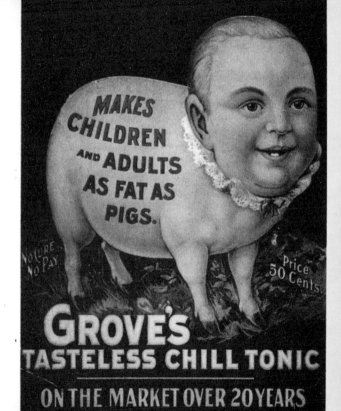

mail order and promotion were key to his scam. Wells would advertise heavily, hoping to lure in patients with his promises – 'I can cure cancer at home without pain, plaster or operation. I have discovered a new and seemingly unfailing remedy for the deadly cancer' ran the spiel for his product, Radol. Upon writing, enclosing $15, a bottle of the miraculous 'radiotized fluid' would be despatched. If a prospective client didn't place an order, they would be bombarded with fliers enticing them to buy at reduced prices; first $10, then $5, then a bargain $2.50. Patients who had the temerity to request a diagnosis before parting with their cash would receive by return a pre-printed form letter from the quack, solemnly declaring he was convinced they had cancer of some part of their anatomy, the exact spot being typed in a blank space especially left for the purpose. Wells made a fortune, and was estimated to be taking in a whopping $70,000 a year when the authorities took an interest in his activities. Procuring some samples of Radol, analysis revealed that they contained no more radioactivity than bath water. In a flourish of quackish showmanship, however, Wells had added a substance that gave a bluish phosphorescent glow to the liquid, which he claimed proved radiation was present.

Another quack, Dr Bye, in 1898 sold a combination of oils to be rubbed into the skin as a cure for cancer. Claiming that he had discovered a method for removing 'every vestige of the cancer virus', patients were asked to fill in a special form detailing their symptoms. The doctor would then prescribe, by return of post, the correct combinations of oils to cure them, a task little short of miraculous considering the oils were made from everyday non-cancer-curing materials like Vaseline, talcum powder, sugar and clay. Various Dr Byes

The 1904 Toxo-Absorbent Cancer Cure was marketed as the 'the most successful cure for cancers ever discovered'. Internal and external cancers, nothing was beyond its reach, incredible when its formulation involved such powerful ingredients as milk, sand, charcoal and witch-hazel leaves. Billing itself as the 'Great Drugless Treatment', it was banned from sale in 1908.

peddled the cancer cure around the country in a fraternal scam; one, B.F Bye, advertised his offices as a grand-looking premises. The building was in fact the local hotel and nothing to do with him.

One way to avoid expensive medical school fees is not to bother going. Showing commendable ambition, the Mixer family declared themselves doctors, but dispensed with the formality of actually attending medical college or taking any instruction. Setting themselves up in business as a father and son medical dynasty around 1900 in the US, they soon launched on to the market their eponymous cancer cure. Advertised with a heart-rending, although entirely fictional, account of Mixer Snr's battle and eventual cure from cancer, the 'Drs' could provide sworn statements from 'Doctors, Lawyers, Mechanics, Ministers, Laboring Men and Bankers' testifying to the efficacy of their cure. A fraud order was issued against them around 1910.

One of the weirdest cancer cures was the Radio-Sulpho treatment. This involved the application of radio-sulphate solution to a cancerous area, and then smearing on a poultice of 'real imported' Limburger cheese! This apparently worked as a magnet on the cancers, drawing them out. But those who were weak ought to be wary, warned the adverts – 'a person that has a weak constitution . . . should never use the

Limburger cheese for a poultice, as it is too powerful'. What cheese was suitable for the frail was never made explicit; a mild Edam perhaps?

Alive and Well

Cancer quackery hasn't disappeared into the past with medicine shows, patent medicines and bogus institutes. Instead the market for strange cures and bizarre remedies has actually grown, driven by the increasing incidence of the disease in its many forms, and the rejection of conventional treatments offered by the medical establishment. Some people prefer to explore alternative treatments for their cancers, with particular methods attracting a fervent following. Others, whom mainstream medicine has failed to help, can fall prey to quacks as they desperately search for a cure. With so many people looking for different ways of curing themselves, it is all too easy for a conman (or woman) to set up in business offering hope and 'medicine' to these people. If it seems that everything gives you cancer, it also appears that almost anything will be hawked as a cure. For all the twentieth-century quacks and cures that have come and gone, some of them had a huge influence.

Harry Hoxsey is one figure around whom debate still murmurs quietly in the health food shop. Born in 1901 he claimed to have inherited a cancer cure handed down to him through his family, although his story changed over the years. His grandfather had 'discovered' the remedy when his favourite horse had a tumour on its leg. Put into a new field when the disease was noticed, Hoxsey's grandfather was astonished to note that over a few months the cancer receded, eventually disappearing completely. The horse was never entered for the Kentucky Derby, but if it had it would no doubt have won, so miraculous was this recovery. Intrigued (no doubt by the prospect of making pots of cash) he investigated further and found that the grass on which the horse had grazed was full of unusual flowers, herbs and roots. Taking his pestle and mortar, grandfather Hoxsey experimented with the assorted flora until he came up with the cancer cure that he was to pass on to his son, Harry's father. When he died of cancer in 1919 (the family remedy oddly failing to cure him), Harry Hoxsey inherited the cancer formula and decided to market it by himself, despite being sued by his siblings for joint ownership and profits. Soon Hoxsey had acquired a reputation for his alternative treatments, showcasing testimonials from people he claimed had been cured by his patent remedy. This soon brought him into conflict with the medical authorities, and a series of court battles raged between Hoxsey and the American Medical Association, who maintained he was a charlatan. The trouble with him, said the authorities, was that he wouldn't supply any evidence of his cures other than florid accounts of miraculous cures from people he had successfully treated; the establishment, countered Hoxsey, was corrupt and self-interested, and didn't want his cure ruining their private party with the big drugs companies. Despite this opposition, by the 1950s Hoxsey had opened a chain of clinics and was treating thousands of patients a year with his methods. There were two different treatments available: a burning paste to be rubbed on to cancers externally, and a internal remedy, which was drunk. A fast-talking Texas salesman, Hoxsey made an absolute fortune, and allied himself to right-wing, UFO-believing evangelist G.B. Winrod and the isolationist, anti-vaccination American Rally.

Hoxsey was dubbed 'the worst cancer quack of the century', in the 1940s. But by the 1970s the surge in interest in natural and herbal remedies meant that his cures started to be reappraised. A documentary film was made, portraying him as a folk hero ruthlessly hounded by the medical establishment. Strangely, analysis of his remedies showed that some of the ingredients he used do have cancer-beating properties, although it didn't show why avoiding pork, tomatoes and vinegar was so important to his cure.

But even with such stalwart allies Hoxsey was a hunted man. In 1957 a judgement against him in court meant that posters – 'Public Beware' – warning of the futility of his cures began to appear against him. By 1960 the last Hoxsey clinic in the USA closed, and the operation fled to Tijuana, Mexico, where it was run by his chief nurse as the Bio Medical Center. (It is still treating patients today.) Hoxsey himself stayed in Dallas, where he dabbled in the oil business. In 1967, he developed prostate cancer. He took his own tonic, but, ironically, it didn't work for him. Although surgery is fairly routine for prostate cancer, he refused to have it, fearing that the Dallas doctors would take their revenge on him on the operating table. Hoxsey spent his last seven years as an invalid, dying in isolation, nearly forgotten. He was buried around Christmas in 1974, without an obituary or tribute in the Dallas newspapers.

Everything's Better

Medical science can now relax, slip out of its white coat and into something more comfortable, safe in the knowledge that all the problems of ill health have been taken care of.

A TURN FOR THE WORSE

Responsible for this leap forward in human understanding is one 'Dr' Hulda Clark, author of the modestly titled *Cure for all Cancers*, and the all-encompassing *Cure for all Diseases*. Curiously these earth-shattering revelations have not met with the publicity you would expect to attend such grandiose assertions. A closer look at the small print perhaps reveals why. The source of most illness, including cancer and AIDS, according to Dr Clark, is parasites and toxins, which wreak havoc on the body. Treatment is as unique as this theory: the parasites and toxins must be expelled through a regime of diet, oral hygiene and two devices called the Syncrometer, used to test for disease, and the Zapper for electrocuting those pesky parasites. Both are actually simple electrical devices unlikely to cure much of anything, although the doctor herself claims that cancer will be cured in five days, regardless of the type or severity. Zappers, including the state-of-the-art Multi-Zap-Zapper, can be purchased from Dr Clark's son ($75 with a money back guarantee if not entirely satisfied), who also kindly endorses them with a certificate so you can be sure that you're not just buying a useless piece of junk sold by a charlatan. Perhaps not surprisingly, Dr Clark has encountered legal difficulties during her time in practice, but fortunately has avoided incarceration. She operates a successful clinic, like the Bio Medical Center, conveniently situated just out of the reach of the US law's arm over the border in Tijuana, Mexico, something of a mecca for strange treatments. Pursued by anti-quack organisations, who campaign to expose the uselessness (as they see it) of her cures, she has attracted a militant following who believe that she has found the key to curing cancer. Quack? The medical establishment definitely think so, but who's to say she's not right? After all, doctors used to think washing their hands between patients was a dangerous idea.

One tumour-busting method that smacks of quackery is psychic surgery. This method claims to remove tumours without leaving a skin wound. The 'surgeon' appears to delve into the human body with his bare hands, coming up with a piece of tissue – the tumour – and leaving no mark on the patient's body. Still practised in Brazil and the Philippines, close investigation has revealed it as a con-trick. A false finger or thumb is used to store the red dye that appears as blood, and an animal organ, soaked in the dye, is hidden in the palm of the surgeon's hand before the operation commences, to later reappear as the 'tumour'.

Everything Gives You Cancer

It is no wonder, though, that quacks are attracted to cancer when there is a constant bombardment of scare stories about how everyday objects can give you cancer. Few realise the danger they risk when they spread margarine (hydrogenated oils, linked to some cancers) on burnt toast (full of hetero-cyclicamines, carcinogens). Feeling depressed about your health? Exposure to the sun's rays may improve your state of mind, but those ultraviolet solar rays can be deadly. Comfort eating won't just add the pounds and put a strain on the heart. Any foods worth eating (i.e. processed fatty foods, glistening with oil, sugar and salt which we are genetically programmed to find delicious), washed down with great gulps of booze, will, upon reaching the stomach, start conspiring together to mutate your cells. Even 'good' foods are at it – broccoli, fish, nuts and other fruit and veg simultaneously contain cancer-preventing and promoting chemicals. Travel will increase your cancer risk (fumes from fuel) so it's probably best to stay at home. Isn't it? Probably not, as the chemicals in carpets, wall paints and household cleaning products can all contain carcinogenic agents. Tap water can contain cancer-causing metals and pollutants. A simple slice of bread may harbour acrymalide, a carcinogen found in baked foods. Flying in an aeroplane increases the likelihood of exposure to radiation at altitude. Speaking on a mobile telephone may increase the risk of some cancers. Even gardening is fraught with risk, with all that deadly radon leaking from the soil.

This list could be virtually endless, but then again so could the list of cancer cures currently available. From existing solely on a diet of grapes, to eating the processed pits of apricots (used in the controversial cancer drug Laetrile), there are literally thousands of cures available, from the pseudoscientific to the downright strange. Electromagnetic scanning for cancer (perfected, incidentally, by a man who fraudulently claimed he could run trucks with water as fuel) available from a clinic in, you guessed, Mexico, is at the high end of bogus treatments. At the other end are the miscellaneous 'natural' cures like coffee enemas, not wearing synthetic fibres, chewing every mouthful fifty times, drinking urine (your own), and countless herbal remedies and salves. Old Native American Indian recipes, strange teas used by the Incas and Druidical medicines are all obtainable. Like Harry Hoxsey's herbal cure, there may indeed be some benefit against cancer in some of these concoctions. But even if there is, the fact that they are aggressively marketed to vulnerable people does little to help them shed their aura of the medicine show 'miracle cure'; good for making a quick buck, but not much else. Caveat emptor.

A Plague on all Doctors

When one of the four horsemen of the Apocalypse rides into town, dismounts and checks into the local hotel under the name 'Mr Plague', then it's time to worry. Times of plague and pestilence are times of panic and mayhem, the normal rhythm of society is disrupted and the old order goes out of the window. Rich and poor are suddenly equals; the plague is egalitarian and will call at anyone's house. In the great plagues, people would revert to old superstitions and wild remedies in an attempt to avoid infection or find a cure. If most of the population saw the plague as the divine wrath of God visited upon their miserable heads, there was one sector of society that positively welcomed the news of contagion. Anticipating soaring profits and outstanding quarterly figures, nothing guaranteed a quack good trade like a nice outbreak of plague.

In terms of medical practice, it was hard to separate quacks and mainstream physicians by their plague treatments. Theories abounded about what caused the plague, and how

Part of the trouble with plague was that no one knew what caused it. One theory was that it was caused by miasmas – bad air. There would certainly been a lot of this about, with people slinging the contents of their chamber pots into the street, animals and rotting vegetables everywhere and general hygiene pretty low down the list of civic priorities. Other popular causes were an infelicitous alignment of the planets, and divine retribution. In fact there were two types of plague, with two separate methods of infection: *pnuemonic* plague was spread by infected people and carried on the air – the coughs and sneezes of a plague-ridden person could be fatal if inhaled. *Bubonic* plague was spread by the bite of fleas which travelled on the infected *rattus rattus* – the black rat. The disease resulted in huge boil-like swellings on the lymph nodes, the feared buboes.

it could be treated. Quacks were perhaps more eager to cry up their wares in handbills than 'legitimate' doctors, but in some neighbourhoods it was all that was available; in the great plague in London in 1665, for example, many doctors and physicians fled to the country to avoid infection, leaving the city-dwellers to whatever treatments they could still find.

Patent remedies and cures were available by the dozen, but it was a risky career choice to carry on selling direct to a pestilential public. Daniel Defoe in his *Journal of the Plague Year* noted that an 'abundance of them died', and Samuel Pepys recorded in his diary that only one apothecary was left alive in Westminster after a few months of plague. Physicians of any kind had to weigh up the profits to be made treating plague victims against the potential loss of their own lives.

Quacks peddled specific plague medicines – 'anti-pestilential pills', 'a universal remedy for the plague', 'sovereign cordial against the corruption of the air', for example – and Defoe noticed that many made great play of their experience in dealing with plagues in other cities, like the 'High German Doctor' who had, while residing in Amsterdam, 'cured multitudes of people that actually had the plague upon them'.

These unlikely CVs lured massive amounts of trade to the doors of the quacks, who would also try to snare people using the old ploy of advertising that consultations and

 The pub business diversified into the plague medicine market. Drinkers at the Green Dragon tavern in Cheapside could buy an anti-plague pint. At sixpence a time this was an expensive drink by anyone's standards in 1665.

One effect of the plague was to make people cast about for someone to blame. The Jews were a popular scapegoat, and in an outbreak of plague in Strasbourg in 1348 20,000 were massacred, accused of poisoning the well water.

advice were free to the poor. The advice was free, it was true, but invariably recommended that the patient needed some of the quack's own nostrum, which was only available for hard cash.

Established medicine didn't have much to offer in the way of plague treatment either. The Royal College of Physicians endorsed the use of roasted onions, stuffed with figs and treacle and pressed against the buboes as a method of cure. Toads were especially sought after in times of plague. A toad simmered in milk was one remedy, and the powder of dried toads was used in various medicines. One cure recommended a dead toad, dried out over a fire. The shrivelled amphibian was then pressed against a swollen buboe, where it would draw the infection out and into its own desiccated corpse.

Doctors of the time, like their counterparts in previous plague outbreaks across Europe, took to wearing bizarre clothing designed to guard them against infection. Clad in

For those who could afford it, a unicorn's horn, powdered and combined with other ingredients, was the medicine of choice. Due to the rarity of such creatures, only the extremely wealthy could afford to buy this type of remedy. Elizabeth I owned a unicorn horn that had cost her a reputed £10,000, enough to buy a country estate with a castle.

heavy leather dresses to offer protection, and tottering around on shoes with built-up soles to prevent treading on infected material, doctors carried a white stick with which to beat away infected people who were roaming the streets. They also wore bizarre hoods, which made them look like grotesque birds; the huge beaks were stuffed with aromatic spices and herbs, and the blank eye sockets were covered in thick glass, all to keep the infectious air – the miasmas – from getting in.

To prevent plague all sorts of strange precautions were employed. In Italy during a fourteenth-century outbreak of the Black Death, the authorities fired cannons into the air in an attempt to frighten off the contagion, a practice that found favour with municipal bodies. Even as late as the nineteenth century, this 'cure' was attempted when yellow fever came to America and the colonies. In 1348 the Black Death killed about a third of the population of England and led to the King, Edward III, issuing instructions to the Mayor of London on how to run a plague-free city: 'You are to cause the city to be cleaned from all bad smells, so that no more people will die from such smells.' Meanwhile, in Avignon, the Pope avoided the Black Death by sitting next to a blazing fire all summer.

In plague-ridden times state of mind was an important factor in preserving health. Advice from the fourteenth century insisted that no man should let his thoughts dwell upon death – instead all his thoughts should be, 'directed to pleasing and agreeable and delicious things'. Inspiring landscapes and garden vistas were to be contemplated, and melodious music played at every opportunity. Finally, the contemplation of gold and precious stones was beneficial as it was 'comforting to the heart'.

Other recommendations included: residing in a house sheltered from the wind, with the windows closed; carrying a nosegay of flowers and herbs, frequently inhaling their aromas; eating no poultry, waterfowl or beef; never sleeping in the daytime; striking fish from the menu; avoiding too much exercise, thought injurious to health; never cooking anything in rainwater, or olive oil – 'Olive oil with food is deadly' – and never, ever, bathing. In 1665 London residents subscribed to a variety of preventative measures. Working on the theory that miasma was the route of infection, powerful smells were widely employed to halt the disease in its tracks.

Fumigation was popular, and people lit smelly fires to prevent infection, sometimes using dangerously volatile materials; gunpowder was burnt and guns discharged. Bedclothes were aired over smoking fires, and brimstone and saltpetre were favourite fumigants. Doctors recommended fumigation should take place twice daily. With the plague ravaging the city, fires being lit and gunshot whistling around, London wasn't a safe place to be. Treacle was a well-respected plague antidote, and came in a variety of flavours, from Venetian treacle to London treacle 'n' rue. One man recommended that keeping a gold coin in the mouth, especially those from the reign of Elizabeth, was effective against the plague when out walking amongst the sick.

Vinegar sales shot up in 1665. As a strong-smelling substance it was highly valued. Letters were always aired over vinegar before being sent to remove from them all possible infection. Daniel Defoe reported one woman who would wash her head in vinegar, and even snort it up her nose if the air was particularly bad.

A TURN FOR THE WORSE

Some people tried to catch syphilis, believing this would protect them from the plague.

Smoking was also thought to prevent the plague and children as young as three were encouraged to smoke. Boys at Eton were flogged for failing to smoke at the time of the great plague.

When the plague was effectively ended by the fire of London in 1666, Daniel Defoe noted that although the people returned to the city from the countryside where they had sat the contagion out, quacks were slow to return. Was it because many of them had ended up in the vast burial pits that surrounded London, or was it because, perhaps, the uselessness of their cures and their avaricious exploitation of sick people were not fondly remembered by those who had survived?

SEXUAL HEALING

The stigma of venereal disease made it an excellent field for the shadier sort of medical practitioner to establish a lucrative practice. A quick glance round a waiting room filled with the afflicted would reveal one shared symptom: shame. Embarrassment and fear of discovery provided an ideal constituency for unscrupulous quacks to exploit. Not only would their patients be willing to pay top prices to be rid of their disease, but their awkward predicament also left them deprived of any patient rights. It was possible to sell them an expensive and ineffective cure, for what recourse did they have? Very little, because to complain would be to reveal the shameful secret of their condition, and expose them to the gossip and ridicule of their friends and neighbours. This made the treatment of VD much more profitable than, say, tooth drawing; after all someone might warn you off a certain barber-surgeon by showing you the mess they had made of their gums, but they would hardly be likely to drop their trousers and wave their blighted member about in warning of a rogue pox-doctor.

Fear of venereal disease was widespread, and from the 1500s a flourishing industry grew around it. Although syphilis (the 'pox') wasn't the only rash in town, it was the most feared and subsequently the most lucrative. Always eager to blame a foreigner for their problems, for centuries people had pointed accusingly at other nationalities as being the bringers of infection. To the French it was the Italian or Neapolitan pox, while to the Italians it was the French disease. Germans blamed it on the Poles and vice versa, with Britain and Spain agreeing with the Italians that it was down to the 'mangy' French, widely accepted as being slovenly in their linen. Everyone else blamed Turkey. Myths abounded about how it was spread, and Gideon Harvey in his 1678 book *Little Venus unmask'd* listed a few of them: it was a confusion of the planets that gave rise to the disease, said some, while others held that sex between a leper and a prostitute had engendered the whole thing. Nonsense, said another group, who had heard first-hand that the Spanish had put leper's blood in the wine in Greece to infect billeted troops. 'The Germans,' sneered Harvey, 'were of the opinion that feeding too oft upon Pease and Bacon might breed the pox, and therefore their magistrates forbad the selling of all sorts of

Sailors were widely held to be responsible for spreading syphilis, bringing back the infection from their jaunts abroad to the fleshpots of Europe. William Buchan, a doctor who had made venereal disease a profitable speciality, reported being consulted by a sailor who had weighed anchor in many a port and who 'was too complete a tar to pay any attention to his health'. Blithely ignoring one's well-being could be fatal, however, warned Buchan, telling of a consultation with a syphilitic patient 'half of whose whole face was eaten away and part of the brain laid bare'.

Peas. This opinion,' he concluded, 'is so unreasonable that it needs no confutation.' More plausibly, many people blamed seafarers returning from abroad.

With morbid fear of contracting venereal disease rife, the doctors of seventeenth- and eighteenth-century London could hardly put a foot wrong, and cures and products flooded the market. Newspapers and handbills hawked various potions: 'Glad tidings to all unfortunate venereal patients', began one, with avuncular directness. Popular cures like the Balm of Gilead were sold for great profit and purported to be made from rare and mythical substances. In this case the inventor claimed 'seeds of gold' discovered by alchemists were the key ingredient. Hawked as a cure for the pox, it in fact was mostly flavoured brandy, with James Boswell (1740–95) an enthusiastic customer. Another medicine Aqua Mirabilis was supposed to combat not only VD, but the plague, dropsy and palsy as well. It was, in fact, a load of manure – quite literally. The main ingredient was dried horse dung mixed with oil. Velno's Vegetable Cure was popular, sold in Europe and the New World despite satirists' warnings that it would turn patients' limbs into plants. Other remedies included Bateman's Drops for venereal complaints, Leake's Genuine Pills – 'much used for effectually curing the Venereal disease in a short time' – and Restorative Electuary, a 'sovereign remedy for venereal complaints'. For those who feared that they may have come unstuck 'sporting in the Garden of Venus', as one handbill put it, helpful guides to spotting symptoms were circulated by doctors and apothecaries alike. Lurid descriptions of scabs, buboes, 'running at the reins' (a watery discharge from the penis, charmingly referred to as 'gleet') and swellings of the groin were guaranteed to make any rake wonder whether they ought to invest in a precautionary pill and tincture. By including more vague, general complaints in the list of warning signs anyone with aches, pains, itches and mouth ulcers found themselves wondering if they too hadn't somehow come by an unfortunate infection. Aware that many people would be loath to be seen at the clap-doctors or the apothecary's shop, some enterprising quacks offered a consultation by post scheme, where you despatched a few guineas and a bottle of urine off to the doctor, and he sent you back his diagnosis and his patent remedy. In London in the eighteenth century, doctors realised that potential patients suffering from the 'lues venera' were shamefaced about consulting with them in the broad light of day. Not wanting to lose out on a potential source of revenue, the quacks soon hit upon the idea of staying open late at night so their pox-ridden clients could visit them under cover of darkness. Their advertisements and handbills would proclaim that they were open all hours, and often contained details of which configuration of lighted candles in the window signalled the doctor's establishment. Some enterprising practitioners also offered secret or concealed entrances to their consulting chambers, enabling undetected visits to be made.

Symptoms

Scabs, running sores and other signs of loose living were all signs which pointed the path to the doctor's door. Harvey listed the early warning signs, which could easily be confused with scurvy: dusky pimples, pains, retching and fever. These would progress swiftly on to more troubling developments: 'rottenness' of the bones, consumption, a 'pocky running at the reins' and, in some cases, a man's 'yard' being eaten away by the disease. A helpful Q&A was published, which offered information to those who wanted to know more, including topics such as: What part of the body would be worst affected (the 'secret' parts); how far the pox could travel ('pocky steems can only be transmitted a hand's breadth'); and if too much sex could give you the pox (yes).

Treatment

But even if you did somehow manage to conceal from your nearest, if evidently not dearest, your poxed state, it would be very difficult to carry on hiding it once treatment began. The main remedy for syphilis at the time was mercury, and it was conspicuous in it's effects on patients. Common side effects of mercury treatment were fever, sweating, excessive salivation, loose teeth, a bleeding mouth and a permanent fetid stench emanating from the patient. One seventeenth-century sailor who attended a doctor while on leave was prescribed mercury pills. Upon taking them, noted the physician, he was seized by a violent discharge of blood and saliva from his mouth 'so as to fill several wash-hand basins'. Such reactions to so poisonous a substance were common, and many people with venereal disease from medieval times to the Victorian era lived in fear of the cure as much as the disease itself.

Mercury had been an established medicine since the fourteenth century, but its devastating effects were well known, and the accounts of his own syphilitic suffering by German scholar and knight Ulrich von Hutten (1488–1523) paint a grim picture. Treatments were brutal. Patients would be taken to small steam rooms – 'stews' – for twenty or thirty days at a time. Seated or lying, they were smeared with a mercury-based paste, swathed in blankets and left to sweat it out. Mucus and bloody gunge poured from their mouths, gums and noses, and sores sprouted on tongues, cheeks and lips. Teeth fell out, and everybody stank of rotting flesh.

Von Hutton gloomily reported that one man killed three patients in a day by overheating the stew – the belief that the hotter it was the sooner they would be cured proving to be a deadly mistake. The patients couldn't bear the temperature and died.

Other people perished from suffocation caused by swollen throats restricting their breathing. Mercury could also be taken by mixing it into pills, it could be injected (sometimes directly into the penis), and it was available as a tincture to drink. There were even reports that one entrepreneur made mercury-coated underpants to allow the wearer to enjoy the benefits of constant application throughout the day directly on to the diseased parts. Mercury cures were produced in different specifications, depending on the patient's symptoms. The Hermaphroditick cure involved mercury pills and antimony pills, whereas the Herculean cure involved using great force against the disease by means of promoting massive salivation in the patient. For desperate cases, only the Gigantean cure would do, although this came with the warning that it may be better to hang oneself rather than have to suffer it, consisting as it did of an ointment of mercury, acid and hog's fat applied to the genitals. Some doctors offered secret locations where patients could undergo their treatments (a sort of modern-day Betty Ford clinic) to help avoid detection, but in the main, if you were having a course of mercury treatment, everybody knew about it.

A seventeenth-century cure for the 'Hectic Pox': take one young cock and boil it well with herbs and spices. Also add three ounces of red worms, taken from a horse's dunghill and washed in white wine. Mix together with crushed vineyard snails to make a poultice.

Alternative Medicine

The horrors of such treatments meant that anyone selling a cure for VD that didn't involve mercury was on to a good thing. Some doctors favoured a more hands-on approach. In 1796 a book published about VD, *Observations Concerning the Prevention and Cure of the Venereal Disease*, recommended mere washing of the genitals as the best way to ward off a dose of the clap or worse. The writer demonstrated the success of this technique by giving the example of a man who wanted to pass on his infection to a lady 'with a view to ascertain a point of jealousy', but failed to do so, attributing this to her extraordinary attention to cleanliness. However, washing with water alone wasn't going to make any money for doctors – they needed to sell a preventative if they weren't peddling a cure. Accordingly, various additives for washes were developed, containing anything from honey, lead or turpentine to vinegar. Some gentlemen, it was noted in the book, preferred to use any liquor to hand – beer, punch, wine or even brandy, warmed, if required, by holding it in the mouth first. In perhaps one of the earliest examples of the economy pack, patients buying some lotion to inject into their afflicted members were given enough to help out a few similarly troubled friends. Sufferers were also advised to keep to the straight and narrow when trying to rid themselves of the disease. Food of a stimulating nature was to be avoided, and there certainly wasn't to be any hard drinking or wrestling, both of which could promote a disastrous swelling of the testicles. In this case, the only thing to do was to apply leeches to the scrotum and surrounding parts until the swelling went away. In severe cases laudanum was to be rubbed on to the penis, and the patient bidden to 'avoid the sight of such objects as may excite lascivious ideas'. Patients who had let their whole equipment go to rack and ruin were recommended to use *bougies* (curved pieces of metal) to keep everything open and at least working in some fashion. The book concluded its advice with a dire tale about a man who had to clear his passage with a knitting needle every time he wanted to urinate.

Lighting the Fire

Of course, it wasn't all about treating disease. There was also the business of selling remedies for better sex and increased potency, and this wasn't solely the preserve of doctors. Witches, wise women and healers all had their warty hands on sex, long before the quacks got in on the act. Folk remedies advocated stoking up the lusty fires in women by giving them sage or mandrake root. Pre-Viagra, men who needed to stiffen the sinew could by chewing ash seeds or eating mint.

Daisies applied to the gonads were supposed to lower the libido, while Nicholas Culpeper, proving that man shares no

In a move that would horrify gum-chewing troops everywhere, soldiers were briefly forbidden mint in case it inspired them to make love, not war.

genetic material with rabbits, believed lettuce 'abate[d] bodily lust'. Those suffering from a dose of the clap were advised to nestle their organ in the warm innards of a freshly killed fowl.

Dr Sex

Dr James Graham can probably be called the greatest quack (1745–1794). His genius rested on his early recognition that sex sells. He enjoyed a career as the premier sexual authority of the age, aided by his astute eye for a marketing opportunity and innate showmanship. His early career took him to the USA where a meeting with Benjamin Franklin alerted him to the possibilities of electrical medicine. Returning to Europe, full of his belief in electricity or 'celestial fire' as a wonder cure, he practised as a doctor in various places, building up a list of clients who were well placed in society. The medical treatments he practised were certainly radical, forcing them to sit on electrified thrones while he pumped a charge through them, or making them squat in electrical baths eating his patent 'aetherial' medicines. Still, his patients seemed to enjoy all this, and, encouraged, Graham decided to try his luck in London. In 1780 he proudly opened his 'Temple of Health' in the Strand, advertising 'The Magnificent Electrical Apparatus and the supremely brilliant and Unique decorations of the Magical Edifice of this enchanting Elysian Palace!'. Employing costumed men to walk round London drumming up publicity, Graham cannily emphasised the sexual nature of the temple with its focus on beauty, youth, vigour and procreation. It also helped that he put on a daily show where the 'gentlemen of the rosy rod' would bring in a semi-clad young girl representing the goddess of health, upon whom Graham would demonstrate the benefits of the temple using her body as an example. This was all arousing stuff, and people flocked to the temple to pay their entrance fee and catch a look at some bare flesh. Upon arrival, and after handing over their two shillings, punters were able to admire the opulent surroundings designed to stimulate the senses. Erotic pictures, music, scents and beautiful assistants lounging around all added to the sensual atmosphere Graham was trying to create. The walls were decorated with crutches, sticks, eyeglasses and other medical paraphernalia, which had supposedly been left behind by patients who had been cured in the temple. For an extra fee, the upstairs of this palace of health was available for viewing, where various electrical machines, fizzing and sparking away with celestial fire and ready to invigorate the pallid and the wan for a suitable sum, were displayed.

Graham also had his own line of specially designed products. Available in quantities to suit any pocket, the public were able to choose from a range of medicines that covered most eventualities, especially in matters libidinous. Nervous Aetherial Balsam, a kind of early Viagra, promised to restore worn-out constitutions and guaranteed procreation. Electrical ether was recommended as sniffable protection against the teeming germs of London, while Imperial Pills would cleanse and purify the blood, a prerequisite for successful lovemaking. A daily dose of these remedies would set up the puniest and weakest of persons, if they could afford it, particularly those who were suffering from performance difficulties, or were having problems generating offspring. Also available was a range of books, sold in discreet brown wrapping and probably best described as medico-porn, the most popular of which was *Private Advisers* – concerning the boudoir antics of ladies and gentlemen of quality, for discreet delectation.

High Voltage

But for those who came to the Temple of Health not just to gawp at the show, and for whom a handful of pills and a stimulating book were not enough, the good doctor offered other treatments, based on electricity. By far and away the most exciting of these, and the centrepiece of Graham's whole enterprise, was the Grand Celestial Bed, a fertility shrine made powerful by magnetism and 'electrical fire'. Available for hire for a '£50 bank note' (a massive sum at the time), couples who used the bed would not only enjoy astonishing 'superior ecstasy', but also guaranteed conception after a night of supercharged sex. 'The barren must certainly become more fruitful when they are powerfully agitated in the delights of love, claimed Graham. Accessed from a private entrance on to the street, the bed was an impressive 108 feet square, and stood upon twenty-eight pillars of glass. Above was a dome, filled with odoriferous spices and herbs, which were to provide invigorating wafts over customers, and decorated with statues that played music via a hidden organ. At the head of the bed, sparking with electricity, was the great first commandment of the Temple: 'Be Fruitful, Multiply and Replenish The Earth'. If this didn't provide enough excitement for any especially lacklustre clients, the bed could also revolve on its axis and tilt like a bucking bronco. The mattress was stuffed with either hay, or sometimes (no doubt for the very discerning), the hair from the tails of English stallions, renowned for its springiness and elasticity.

This bed generated huge publicity for Graham, and the Celestial Bed became the talk of London. Rich men and lords willingly coughed up the necessary cash to enjoy a night

One of the 'goddesses' of the temple was a young Emma Lyon, who began her career in the Temple of Health demonstrating an unusual remedy, which involved sporting naked in a mud bath, to the delight of assembled onlookers. She later became the plaything of various luminaries of the day before ending up as Lady Hamilton, Nelson's mistress.

enjoying the stimulating pleasures it offered, not always with their wives. It was rumoured that, for a fee, it might be possible to hire both the bed and one of the handmaidens from the Temple of Health, enabling Graham to extract even more cash from his public.

However, after a while, bookings fell away, and the Temple of Health moved to a cheaper premises in Pall Mall and became the Temple of Hymen. Admission rates were halved, and use of the Celestial Bed was slashed to £25 a night to boost profits. The temple also became a gambling den. Undeterred, Graham made sure that there was still plenty on offer to tempt people through the doors. New and more complicated electrical machinery was brought in, which sparked and crackled ever more impressively, and the lectures on health, which had previously been delivered by Graham himself, were instead given by junior priests of the temple each afternoon and evening, leaving Graham free to promote his other great medical hobby horse besides electricity – earth bathing. A firm believer in this practice, he recommended patients regularly indulged in mud baths or 'earth soaks'. This, he claimed, would ensure longevity, with 100 or even 150 years of age being the reward of the diligent soil bather. To this end he had pits dug in the floor of the Temple of Hymen where people could be buried up to their necks, sometimes for hours on end. Those who could not make the time to be buried could at least strap a turf to their chest using 'fresh, icy cold earth brought from the top of Hampstead Hill' if at all possible. Clean and decent living and a healthy, moderated diet were also recommended, and when the temple finally closed in 1784 (bad debts, creditors and Newgate prison all figured in the decision), Graham went on the road extolling the virtues of a simple life and mud bathing. Hard beds, open windows, fresh air, and early hours were all part of the recipe for health, with bathing especially important, something with which his contemporary, the preacher and medical experimenter John Wesley, agreed.

Graham abandoned his earlier adherence to all things electric, but perhaps unsurprisingly retained his bevy of 'goddesses of health' to assist him in live displays of mud bathing. In these he and one of his beautiful assistants would strip naked and be buried up to their necks in mud, whereupon Graham would deliver a lecture describing the invigorating effects in graphic enough detail to bring blushes to the cheeks of ladies in his audience. As time passed, James Graham increasingly cast off his old, quackish ways and became something of a religious zealot, forming the New Jerusalem Church (he was the only member) and trusting entirely to the healing power of nature for all medical needs. Increasingly erratic, he would strip off in the street and give his clothes away, or remain buried in mud, fasting for days on end. He eventually died in 1794 from starvation, having foolishly taken his own considered medical counsel that food was unnecessary for healthy living. Although he had been a great showman, and without doubt made a healthy pot of money from some pretty doubtful practices, Graham actually believed that at least some of his medical treatments did some good. Ironically, the doctor's (although, to be strictly accurate he never really qualified) use of electricity as a medical tool predicted its use in modern hospitals and his emphasis on healthy living and even total fasting (like the 'breatharian' movement today) wouldn't seem out of place in the modern world.

Lovesickness

Lovesickness was a widely recognised medical complaint in the Middle Ages. Although medicine today might be dismissive of such an idea, or at best diagnose it as some sort of depression and prescribe some pills to perk you up, in earlier times this was a condition with its own distinctive symptoms and cures.

It was important to be able to recognise a case of lovesickness when one came up. It was more common in women than men. Women, being softer hearted, were more susceptible than men, although easier to cure; men, meanwhile, were less likely to suffer from lovesickness but much harder to bring to recovery unless wealthy – these men had softer lives, which meant they had big, soft, womanly hearts. Sufferers were distinguishable to the practised eye by a variety of telltale signs. Fluttering eyelids and an irregular pulse, insomnia, pallor and loss of concentration and appetite were early warning signs that not all was well. An examination of the eyes, the mirrors of the soul, was also recommended. Early diagnosis was crucial as left unchecked, the condition could quickly deteriorate into a much more serious situation. Lust might rage out of control, or the patient could fly into a murderous rage at the sight of a pretty face or weep uncontrollably at the sound of a love ballad. The

Persian physician Rhazes (865–925) even warned that people suffering from lovesickness could turn yellow, or even worse into werewolves and go rampaging through graveyards by the light of the moon.

Evidently not a condition to be taken lightly, it was important that the medical establishment (loosely a collection of monks, scholars, physicians and the odd passing alchemist) understood the causes of lovesickness. Generally this was held to be less to do with actual love itself, but instead a build-up of one of the four humours, which was causing a system imbalance. The culprit in the case of lovesickness was black bile, housed in the spleen and responsible for a melancholic disposition. As it built up, overwhelming the other essential humours in the body, so the severity of the lovesickness got worse, eventually resulting in death or madness.

Once the symptoms and the cause were understood, the problem of a cure presented itself. The Roman physician Galen said that the accepted remedy for lovesickness was to get rid of the excess black bile, and the best way to do this was to have sex, although, oddly, not with the object of the sufferer's affections. Through intercourse the bile would be discharged via the bodily fluids, and the patient would be both relieved and restored to sound health. Galen happily prescribed bouts of sex to those he diagnosed with lovesickness, and even recommended that health-conscious men make love regularly, even if they didn't enjoy it, to keep themselves fit. This cure, however, ran aground on Catholic doctrine as the Church gained influence, casual sex outside marriage being prohibited even in a medical emergency. Chastity for the single and for priests was sacrosanct, despite the grave consequences this could bring to the devout, such as Thomas, Archbishop of York, who died in 1114. Diagnosed with lovesickness he refused the advice of the doctors to indulge in a bout of recuperative lovemaking, and instead passed away as a result, his chastity intact. Apart from highlighting the lack of moral fibre in the modern Church, Thomas's demise also pointed to the lack of alternative cures for this terrible disease. 'Sufferers could try drinking wine, herbal remedies, relaxing baths and reciting poetry by babbling brooks. A French scholar, Bernard of Gordon (1285–1308), recommended more stringent measures including castration, or beating patients 'until they started to rot'. He also recommended aversion therapy, whereby the object of desire was shown in unflattering situations until the would-be lover found himself so appalled that he was thus cured. Taking his lead from Ovid's 'cure for love', Bernard suggested ploys such as making a snaggle-toothed lover laugh, trying unflattering sex positions, visiting your beloved before they had put on make-up and even spying on them in the toilet.

Hysterical Medicine

There was one condition throughout the history of medicine that doctors consistently diagnosed in women: hysteria. While the pharaohs were building their pyramids, Egyptian doctors took time off from embalming to come up with the idea that a special disease afflicted women, although it was Plato who named it hysteria – literally, womb-disease. The theory was that the uterus of women was responsible for a large proportion of the diseases and maladies they suffered. Illness was caused by the womb becoming unhappy by being starved of the two things that made it content – sex and children. This, after all, reasoned the doctors, was what the womb was for, and so it was only to be expected that an unsatisfied uterus was an unhappy one too, liable to wreak disease and havoc in the body.

Different schools of thought emerged. Plato declared the womb an animal in its own right within the body, while Galen believed it to be an inverted scrotum. Despite these differences, there was a consensus on the hazard to health that an unhappy womb could cause. Annoying the womb, a cantankerous beast, could have serious consequences, and it was understood to be able to move about, leaving its usual position near the pelvis and wandering off around the body, fighting with the other organs. It could even rise up to the throat and strangle its host if sufficiently peeved. A happy uterus equalled a healthy woman, and the wise physician prescribed the marriage bed as a cure of first resort. Deprived of sex or conception, the 'hungry' organ would grow violent, first triggering displays of 'hysteria', and then roaming off around the body. If this occurred, then the physician would be forced to attempt to lure it back in to its rightful place before it travelled too far and strangled the patient. To do this, the hands and feet would be bound and the ankles cut to drain off excess blood. With one hand the doctor would waft foul smelling substances under the nose to drive the womb away from the airway, while with the other hand he waved sweet scents and spices round her genitals to lure the organ down to its rightful place. Once it had returned, an expert would quickly bind up the stomach to hold the uterus in place, and the patient would be revived by having her hair plucked out.

Hysterical symptoms were conveniently wide-ranging, allowing doctors to make a diagnosis from symptoms like

Paracelsus thought that hysteria was caused by the womb having a fit and belching out smoke, which poured around the body suffocating the heart.

fainting, nervousness, insomnia, heaviness in the abdomen, spasms, breathlessness and loss of appetite. If in doubt, hysteria was a convenient catch-all for almost any female complaint.

Drawing on Galen's idea of the womb as an inverted scrotum, doctors thought that women had their own 'seed' like men, which, if unsatisfied by intercourse, would build up to dangerous levels and cause hysterical meltdown (the Vagina Syndrome). Medieval drawings of the womb display the scant knowledge about this fearsome and feared organ; pictures show it sometimes shaped like a cat's head, filled with fully formed little people dancing around in happy anticipation of the day of their birth. Others depict it as a seven-chambered vessel; in the three right-hand chambers male children were generated, and on the left-hand 'sinestra' (literally, ill-favoured) side, females were made. The central chamber, of course, produced hermaphrodites.

Manual Labour

Cures for hysteria divided into two main groups from the Ancient World to relatively recent times. One way was to try to satisfy the unruly womb. This was primarily done through sex, doctors like Ambroise Paré declaring in the sixteenth century that hysterical women should 'bee strongly encountered by their husbands'. Regular intercourse for women was thought beneficial: 'Wives are more healthful than widows or virgins, because they are refreshed with the man's seed, and ejaculate their own, which being excluded, the cause of evill [hysteria] is taken away,' wrote Nicholas Fonteyn in 1630. For doctors in Ancient Greece prescribing sex and conception was less of a problem than for their medieval counterparts, the moral climate being somewhat more temperate. The rising influence of the Church with its attitudes towards sex (Thomas Aquinas thought it a beastly business best avoided) forced the medical profession to adopt a more hands-on approach to treatment. Robert Burton (1589–1655) dubbed hysteria 'maid's, nun's and widow's melancholy', and it was these type of women who most needed treatment, said the doctors. Without husbands though, how were the symptoms to be relieved?

The answer was simple. Stimulation. Physicians and midwives had long resorted to rhythmic rubbing of the genitals of hysterical women to bring relief from their symptoms. Such manipulation, noted doctors, resulted in a paroxysm, which seemed to relieve the hysterical symptoms. Recommended by the Egyptians, the Greeks and the Romans, this form of treatment had a long medical history, and was accepted as an effective treatment for 'womb-fury'. Riverius, physician to the King of France (1589–1653) recommended that, 'the genital parts should by a cunning midwife handled and rubbed, so as to cause evacuation of the over-abounding sperm'. Doctors, who quickly became bored with such manual drudgery, prescribed horseback riding, rope climbing and vigorous rocking chairs for the various nuns and virgins who required treatment. Some advocated the use of pessaries made from irritants, which would promote heating and general twitchiness in the nether regions and bring about the release of built-up seed.

The prudish Victorians looked upon hysteria with horror. Identifying it with an ever-widening range of complaints, it was taken up as the popular disease of the age. Rebranded 'neurasthenia', any young, or not so young, woman could find herself diagnosed as hysterical and whipped off for treatment for something as innocuous as holding her own political beliefs. The womb and reproductive organs were still believed to be the cause of hysteria, but the squeamish distaste with which Victorians viewed sex (particularly in females) gave the whole thing a sinister new twist. Hysterical behaviour was a result of disorder and uproar of the female reproductive system, affecting the whole body and leading to mental instability.

Doctors grew famous on the back of their treatments of hysterical females, like Roger Battey. An American surgeon of great repute, Battey became an evangelist for removing a woman's ovaries as a treatment for hysteria after he successfully hauled a 30lb ovarian cyst out of the bloated stomach of the wife of a friend. Convinced that he had not only helped her to wear a corset again, but had also restored her general health, Battey speculated that the ovaries were the seat of anxiety and hysteria. In 1872 he was sent a patient who suffered from convulsions and haemorrhage every month when her period was due. Battey operated to remove her ovaries and after a few shaky days the girl recovered fully, cured of her former ailment. This case caused a sensation and the operation to remove ovaries gained massive popularity amongst doctors. The procedure was even called Battey's operation. As time passed, he began to use this treatment for a widening range of conditions including nervousness, nymphomania, menstrual pain and, ominously, insanity. A new medical term was coined, ovariomania, which was believed to affect women of childbearing years, and any woman displaying neurotic or abnormal behaviour could find herself in line for Battey's operation. Insane asylums in the American south seized upon this idea and scores of women found themselves undergoing needless surgery to remove their ovaries for postnatal depression and epilepsy. Eugenics enthusiasts and racialist groups also took to the idea of ovary removal as a way of guaranteeing racial purity. In 1906 estimates were that in the USA alone over 150,000 women had had their ovaries removed. Around this time the tide began to turn against such ideas; as doctors questioned their scientific basis, Battey's operation was used less and less.

Love Again

If quacks prospered and bizarre theories flourished when medicine and venereal disease met, then a whole new field was opened up when it came to solo sex. Masturbation treatments, male and female, are almost a byword for quackery, although strangely it wasn't really a burning area of interest until about the eighteenth century. Masturbation of women by doctors and midwives for the relief of hysteria was not uncommon, and if patients were cautioned not to do it themselves it was mainly because of the 'doctor knows best' attitude of physicians rather than any fear of contracting disease through self-treatment. Similarly, for men, not much attention had really been paid to this habit. People like Diogenes the Cynic in the fourth century BC merely declared masturbation an effective remedy for the irritation of lust, and of no real significance. However, a major change took place at the beginning of the eighteenth century when in 1710 an anonymous author published a treatise called *Onania, or, the Heinous sin of Self-Pollution and all its Frightful Consequences, in Both Sexes, Considered*. A best-seller, the pamphlet warned against the horrible dangers and risks that masturbation posed, particularly to adolescent males, whom doubtless were its main target. The rewards for practising this 'filthy and odious' habit were many and dreadful. Stunted growth was almost a certainty, and a deformation and withering of the genitals enough to 'render them ridiculous to women' was sure to follow. If, by some chance, a habitual onanist remained robust enough to marry and father children, the offspring would be 'weakly little ones, that either die soon, or become tender, sickly people always ailing and complaining: a misery to themselves, a dishonour to the Human Race, and a scandal to their Parents'. But for the unrepentant self-abuser, or those foolhardy enough to ignore the havoc they wrought upon themselves, the early grave yawned. 'Many Young Men who were strong and lusty before they gave themselves over to this vice,' cautioned the writer, 'have been worn out by it, and . . . without Cough or Spitting, dry and emaciated, sent to their Graves.'

Females who masturbated could expect bouts of a terrible, although unspecified, womb disease and of course the obligatory 'hysterick fits'. Protecting physical beauty was offered as an incentive to desist from this shameful practice: 'It makes 'em look pale, and those that are not of good Complexion, swarthy and haggard.' However, a curious coyness overtook the anonymous author at this point. Rather than detail any more of the calamities that could overtake women who indulged in this practice, he instead deferred to common decency, leaving the reader to draw their own, lurid conclusions, explaining, 'It would be impossible to rake into so much *filthiness*, as I should be oblig'd to do, without offending Chastity.'

Treatment

Happily for those who heeded his warnings and resolved to rid themselves of this vice, the writer also included advice and admonishments on how to achieve a purer state (providing a template for later quacks who would ruthlessly mine this profitable seam). The first thing to be done was to master some kind of mind-control, like the contemplation of 'sad and doleful Objects' to drive out all frivolous and lustful thoughts. Once the imagination had been reined in it was time to pay attention to diet, which was to be so spare as to disappoint even the most devout Puritan. Dry foods and water-gruel were the order of the day. Salted meat (a trigger food, in modern medical parlance, for onanistic behaviour) was forbidden, as was anything that might provoke gas: 'All windy Foods, for the Flatuousness of them, do puff up the Humour . . . And make those parts more turgid; such as Beans and Pease, Artichoaks etc . . .'. The bed was effectively viewed as the masturbator's office, where most business was done. Spending extra time there was extremely dangerous for anyone trying to break the habit. Going to bed with a book on a suitably dull subject was vital, and instead of enjoying a lie-in in the morning, a perilous period for 'your Flesh will be egging you on to sinful Pleasure', springing straight up upon awakening was essential. While asleep, lying only on one side was permitted, and of course, any 'handling of the parts' was prohibited. The instructions concluded with a tip for those young men troubled by nocturnal emissions over which they had no control, which was to spawn a thriving industry in the next century. To prevent 'involuntary Pollutions' tying a loop of string around the neck and attaching it to one's penis before bed ensured that, if any stirrings occurred during the night, the tugging would pull the endangered young man from sleep and allow him deal with the situation before anything serious happened.

Moral Medicine

The influence of *Onania* was huge; no one had ever written such a book before, and the public rushed to buy it. It was also eagerly consumed by other doctors and quack practitioners who were lurking in the undergrowth, and the first of these to get in on the act was a Swiss doctor, Samuel Tissot (1728–97). He produced a thundering condemnation of masturbation, which exceeded that of his anonymous predecessor both in its unbending moral tone and its gruesome medical predictions for the 'sickly weaklings' who had obtained and revelled in this habit. Chief expert on medical hygiene and adviser on plagues to the Pope, Tissot's reputation ensured that his opinions were accorded medical respectability. Tumours, imbecility, blindness, impotence and gonorrhoea, haemorrhoids and death were the rewards of masturbation, he declared. One man he knew of was so addicted to self-abuse that his brain had dried out and could be heard rattling in his head. Most significant was his linking of medical and moral doom, assuring the self-abuser a harvest of torment both in this world and the next, and setting the stage for the increasingly frenzied obsession with stamping out the practice, which was to occupy so many medical minds for the next 150 years.

The Belt and Braces Approach

Increasingly exercised by the spectre of the masturbating youth, the Victorians became obsessed with identifying members of the brotherhood of Onan and preventing them any opportunity to indulge in their reprehensible rites. Sermonising and warnings were replaced with medical interventions designed to stop the practice in its tracks. The talent for engineering that the Victorians demonstrated to such effect in buildings and bridges was responsible for the invention of many new medical devices, amongst which were the stethoscope and surgical anaesthesia. The minds of inventors, medical or otherwise, also turned themselves to the problem of the masturbator, and it wasn't long before 'medical' devices began appearing on the market, promising a solution. Drawing their inspiration from the belt-length of looped string suggested in *Onania*, these devices were designed to alert the incipient masturbator of trouble brewing below, and provide a painful incentive to condition them away from such activities.

Trusses and 'self-protectors' could be worn under clothing, and would stop the wearer acting on any lascivious thoughts as they occurred throughout the day. Albert Todd applied for patents for both an electrically charged cage, which was attached to an special belt and fitted over the genitals, and a solid-steel penis cylinder to 'limit longitudinal extension', delivering a jolt of electricity sufficient to burn flesh upon erection. A Dr Everett Flood wrote in 1888 of his success in treating a patient by encasing his hands in plaster: 'the boy's genitals might have been in the next county for all the sensation his hands could communicate'.

Spermatorrhoea, a term coined for the involuntary and fruitless loss of sperm, was particularly feared by the Victorians. Even if masturbation was curbed, there was still the threat of nocturnal emissions which could gravely affect mental and physical health. Where the Ancient Greeks had slept with lead ingots on their chests to prevent nightly loss, the Victorian first line of defence were devices like Spermatorrhoea rings, toothed cylinders which were placed over the penis, metal spines pointing inwards. Even the slightest tumescence caused pain.

Refinements were added, like pressure plates covered in abrasive materials, but these were somewhat discredited when research found that direct pressure 'served rather to increase them to diminish sexual excitement, thereby tending much more to promote than to prevent the disease which it is designed to cure'. Other devices like Stephenson's Spermatic Truss, a leather and canvas affair strapped to the body, were popular sellers.

Some quacks patented less violent solutions. In 1893 Mr F. Orth developed air and water penile coolers, which worked by detecting any erection and bathing the offending organ in cold water, or submitting it to an icy blast from a fan. Somewhat inconveniently they required the installation of a full plumbing system under the bed. Joseph Lees, calling upon the latest developments in technology in 1900, invented a system where an electrical circuit connected the penis to one of the newfangled gramophone machines. Thus, when the music lover's dreams turned lubricious, the rising baton would start the gramophone playing and they would wake in the darkness to the sound of their favourite concerto.

In 1889 James Bowen brought to market a machine comprising a cap that fitted over the end of the penis, secured by two chains which were clipped into the pubic hair. When the wearer experienced any excitement, the chains would be pulled taut, and the pubic hair given a wrench.

Male castration was also occasionally practised for cases of masturbationary insanity, but was not widely accepted by the medical establishment, perhaps unsurprisingly considering that most doctors (quack and otherwise) were men.

A Woman's Lot

Victorian men seemed to have spent an inordinate amount of time thinking about female masturbation. Linked in their minds with the inherent female disease of hysteria, masturbation, they believed, was bound to aggravate hysterical and nervous illness.

One notorious quack emerged with a treatment, which was designed to nip the problem in the bud. Around 1858, Isaac Baker Brown identified 'peripheral excitement' (a euphemism for masturbation) as the root cause of female illness, mental and physical. In his book *On the Curability of Certain Forms of Insanity*, he described eight different types of female malady in an ascending scale, starting with hysteria through to spinal irritation, three types of fits, idiocy, mania, and finally death. His remedy was simple: clitoridectomy, the surgical removal of the clitoris. Snipping away with his scissors, he mutilated the genitals of scores of Victorian women (often against their will) to 'cure' them of their illnesses. So convinced was he of his procedure, Baker Brown published a self-congratulatory tract

 The Victorians were convinced that foot-treadle-operated sewing machines and bicycles were dangerous devices that encouraged masturbation. Excessive stitching or cycling could even lead to lesbianism.

detailing his cases. Medical opinion was horrified, although possibly more by the boastful tone of his work than by what he was actually doing. Although he was a qualified surgeon, his reputation was soon shredded and he was driven from practice, his methods disappearing with him. Medicine would soon find a very different way of dealing with 'hysterical' women.

Domestic Bliss

Around the end of the nineteenth century, advertisements began appearing in women's magazines that promised a new type of invigorating health treatment. 'TO WOMEN I address my message,' began one in the *National Home Journal*. 'Gentle, soothing, invigorating and refreshing. Invented by a woman who knows a woman's needs.' 'Thrilling, invigorating, penetrating,' enticed another in *Modern Priscilla*. The mystery products in question were 'health' vibrators, sold openly in the popular press. At a time when the public, particularly in the US, were in thrall to new machines and technological advance, the home vibrator marked a new development in the sex medicine market. Doctors had been using mechanical vibrators in their surgeries for years as a way of speeding up the tedious task of manipulating hysterical women under their care to clinical 'paroxysm', a cure that had been around for centuries but was viewed with increasing distaste by fastidious doctors. Instruments like the electrical Chattanooga sold for $200 as medical apparatus, with a variety of vibrational probes and attachments for use on women (and sometimes men, as one medical advert graphically showed). Before this, water-powered, hand- and foot-cranked models had been used, but the spread of the electricity network gave the vibrator market a boost.

The vibrator was the fifth home appliance to be electrified after the sewing machine, the fan, kettle and toaster.

'American Vibrator may be attached to any electrical light socket, can be used by yourself in the privacy of dressing room or boudoir, and furnishes every woman with the very essence of perpetual youth,' claimed an advert in the *Woman's Home Companion*. Other vibrating apparatus like chairs, corsets and belts were also sold on the back of dubious health claims, but the vibrator itself was king of the appliances. Pictures in the magazines showed people vibrating their abdomens or heads with various devices, often blithely ignoring the tangle of flex sparking in a socket inches away. In the end it was the movies that saw the end of the vibrator era, when early stag films revealed the instrument being used in a shockingly depraved way. Suddenly the explicit sexual nature of the machines was all too apparent, and the advertisements vanished from the press, only reappearing in the 1960s in quite a different sort of publication.

Something for Sir?

Quackery and male sexual performance are a perfect match. Anxiety and embarrassment conspire to deliver a patient who will desperately cling to any straw that is offered, however foolish it may appear. A brief tour of the internet today is like walking round a medieval marketplace selling doubtful cures. Mountebanks and charlatans cry their mail-order wares, all designed to increase sexual attractiveness and performance. Dressed up as either cutting-edge science – 'new growth hormone discovered' – or esoteric historical wisdom –

'ancient Chinese remedy used for 'thousands of years – increase your potency AND size' – they are new variants on an old theme.

Sex-related quacks had a field day at the beginning of the twentieth century, with new products being advertised almost every week in the back of newspapers and magazines. Targeted at those who wanted to recapture the lost virility of their youth, an abundance of penile splints, pills, electrical belts and assorted paraphernalia hit the market. Some were pretty straightforward, like the 'wimpus': a rigid splint for the unenthusiastic organ 'an aid for impotents'. There were a variety of similar products: the Erector, the Robot-Man ('if your glands are weak'), the Monster Auto-Man ('when nature fails entirely') and the Saddle ('to assist men in protecting themselves from becoming too old'). Electrical belts, like the Sansom Special, were worn to reintroduce vigour and vitality, often with a specially electrocuted sack to dangle the testicles into. Vacuum pumps did brisk business, promising to 'complete the development of abnormal, undersized parts'. 'It is impossible for a woman to love a man who is sexually weak,' warned the makers of the Perfect Organ Developer. 'It is well-established scientific fact that the musicians, financiers and pugilists are men of exceptionally strong sexual power,' they added, contributing to the woes of the tone deaf, poor pacifists everywhere.

One quack remedy that was particularly notorious was the goat gland cure promoted by 'Dr' J.R. Brinkley. Proud holder of two bogus medical diplomas, the Doc built up a thriving empire selling the surgical implantation of goat's testicles into impotent men, having first carried out the procedure on a farmer who had come to him for help in 1918. The farmer, said Brinkley, was completely cured two weeks after the treatment and had even gone on to have a son christened 'Billy'. Goat gland fever spread quickly, abetted by Brinkley's genius for self-promotion on his own radio station. Selling a variety of his quack medicines via a network of specially chosen pharmacists, he pushed the goat gland cure so successfully that at its peak, sixty goats a week were donating their testicles to pseudo-science. Eventually the authorities caught up with Brinkley. His medicines were revealed to be no more than coloured water, and the goat cure itself was exposed as absolute rubbish.

Another bizarre treatment aimed at increasing men's glandular (and by implication, sexual) health were the prostate gland probes. These were effectively heaters, phallic-shaped, which were inserted into the male rectum to deliver a warming glow to the prostate gland. The manufacturers of the Recto-Rotor Lubricating Dilator backed up their product with an ad campaign that played on male fears of impotence and unsatisfactory performance. Used with a specially designed lubricant, it was essentially inserted to 'furnish a constant heat to the rectal anatomy'. Baseless in their claims, the companies who produced the devices were regularly prosecuted by the authorities during the 1920s and 1930s.

ALL IN THE MIND

Healthy mind, healthy body, said the Romans. But is it wise to take medical advice from a group of people who believed that birthing problems could be avoided if a man paraded a live hare around his wife when she was in labour? Maybe not. But the bizarre remedies for madness and mental illness through history show that the mind or soul was considered just as important as the physical body when attempting a cure. Often the spirit was the first place to which a doctor would refer when diagnosing a mad patient.

Mental illness can take many forms, and the type was usually determined by whatever the healer believed had caused it. Remedies followed accordingly. Therefore, people thought to be mad from demon possession or some such, were most likely to be treated through exorcism, whereas those treated medically, however brutally, were at least thought to have physical, and therefore curable, illnesses. Often, however, the two were mixed up.

ALL IN THE MIND

Madness BC

The belief in evil spirits as a cause of illness and pain was an attempt to rationalise the inexplicable puzzle of illness. If you fell off a log, or stabbed your foot accidentally with your spear, then the cause of the resultant pain was obvious. Mental illness, though, was different. With no visible causes, the only conclusion ancient humans could reach was that it was caused by some sort of malevolent force. The early Hindus believed that when the gods were angered they entered a person and produced mental disease, and doctors used herbs, chanting, and kind, gentle treatment. The brain as the site of mental function, as opposed to the stomach (where many thought the vital spirit resided) was identified by the Ancient Egyptians, and the Persians listed 99,999 diseases in a medical handbook, including mental disturbances, which were caused by demons. The Ancient Chinese thought that deviation from filial responsibilities caused madness, and ceremonies to appease dead ancestors were common. In such times of trouble, the only place to go was the shaman. With a hotline to the spirit world, he would be able to intercede and communicate on behalf of the patient, and, assorted deities willing, effect a cure.

Every early culture had healers or shamans. They were

Shamans were often chosen for the job because they were different, physically. They might have extra toes or fingers, or even be epileptic, which was considered to signal some divine designation, most likely because the frenzied nature of the fits were believed to be an ecstatic spiritual trance. The Ancient Greeks even called it the 'sacred disease'.

QUACK MAGIC

The shaman in ancient African cultures would drip blood from the head of the mad patient on to a young goat, which would then be driven off into the bush to die, carrying with it the evil spirits. This is the origin of the word 'scapegoat' – literally one who takes on the guilt or burdens of others.

part priest, part magician, able to bridge the gap between the earthly realm and the exclusive spirit world. As well as doing odd jobs like summoning rain and locating lost livestock, the shaman carried out medical treatments based on potent herbal brews and exorcism.

However, shamanic treatments were generally limited, and might otherwise involve beating with flaming brands, or stoning and dunking in water to drive off the devils. He also had a nifty line in symbolic cures, such as removing a stone from his mouth when carrying out a treatment, which symbolised the escape of the evil spirits. The patient who had seen this happen would ideally experience relief and immediate freedom from their condition, an early example of the placebo effect. In common with many modern practitioners, his methods were beyond question – 'shaman knows best'. Anthropology has failed to answer the fundamental question of who was truly insane – the shaman who had frenzied fits, saw visions and communed with invisible forces, or the tribesman he was trying to cure.

Exorcism in ancient times was simply achieved by inserting a root up the patient's nose and pulling out the evil spirit. Drawings show it leaving through the nose or mouth.

Need a Doctor like a hole in the head

There were some primitive healers, though, who didn't rely on spiritual methods to cure the mentally ill, although spirits were still often held to be the cause of disease. These early forerunners of the 'proper' physician had their own methods, not just for curing the insane, but also addressing other ailments and wounds. In Ancient Peru and North Africa, trepanation was often applied to liberate the tormenting demons. Holes were drilled in the skull to provide an easy exit for spirits, and skeletons over 5,000 years old have been found with fissures bored deliberately with drills.

Trepanation still has many advocates, perhaps the most vociferous being Dr Bart Hughes, a medical school graduate who discovered he could get high by standing on his head. Surmising that an increased blood supply to the brain was the way to enlightenment, he abandoned his consumption of LSD and mescaline and took up trepanation as the route to higher consciousness. The Dutch authorities took a different view and rewarded Dr Bart with a spell in a lunatic asylum. One person who took his message on board was Joseph Mellen, who attempted unsuccessfully to trepan himself. Unable to complete the operation single-handed, he called

Trepanation is far from consigned to history. In 2000 the BBC reported the story of a British woman who carried out the procedure on herself. The DIY experiment went wrong when she accidentally drilled in too far and damaged her brain membrane. However, the operation was a success she told the film crew: 'I generally feel better and there's definitely more mental clarity.'

up Dr Bart whose offer to assist was regrettably curtailed by the Home Office who refused him entry in to Britain as an undesirable. He instead turned to Amanda Fielding who agreed to help him. So impressed was she with the results (despite Mr Mellen being rushed to hospital during the operation after passing out), that she underwent the procedure herself, and stood for parliament in 1978, eliciting forty votes from the people of Chelsea with her promise of free trepanation for all on the NHS.

Beasts and Kings

Some of the most detailed early accounts of madness are to be found in the Old Testament. Madness was seen as a punishment from God, and Moses warned the Israelites, 'The Lord shall smite thee with madness.' Because their affliction was believed to be of divine origin, the insane were allowed to wander where they pleased, free from harm and acting as a sort of mobile warning against offending heaven. King David even used this to his advantage when fleeing from danger, only to find himself in the city of his enemies. Pretending to be demented he 'let his spittle fall down upon his beard' (frothing is a universally accepted symptom of madness). The authorities, deciding their city had quite enough lunatics already, released him on his way. Another famous biblical lunatic was Nebuchadnezzer, sixth-century BC king of the Babylonians who was driven mad by God for seven years as a punishment for pride. Condemned to wander the fields like a beast, his 'hairs were grown like eagles' feathers, and his nails like birds' claws'.

Middle Ages doctors would later term this condition

lycanthropy. Although it strictly means transformation into a werewolf, it was used pretty much to describe any patient who believed themselves transformed into an animal. Each country had its own version, based on the local fauna. In India people turned into tigers, in South America into jaguars and in parts of Scandinavia into bears. Less glamorously, people could also turn into pigs, cats and dogs. As the belief in werewolves subsided, so did the cases of this type of insanity, although the credulous French persisted in believing that the *loup-garou* was still at large until the nineteenth century when, no doubt, the last one was caught and promptly cooked up in a wine sauce *aux fines herbes*. (Incidentally, return to human form was effected by having your baptismal name shouted three times by a person simultaneously making the sign of the cross.)

The Greeks and the Romans

The Greeks were the first to start thinking about mental illness as a physical problem. But only a small proportion of high-ranking citizens were able to afford doctors who treated in this way, and the majority of people were content to follow the old method of appeasing the gods in return for a cure. In Greek literature, madness almost always foreshadowed some tragic event. The gods were also understood to make insanity jump out of a mad person and into unwary passers-by. Thus the insane were chained up out of the way if thought dangerous, or banished to wander country lanes if not. Most people had to content themselves with visiting shrines and offering sacrifices and tokens if there was any lunacy in the family. Climate forecasts were also eagerly anticipated, not because the weather prophets had any medical lore, but because windy days were understood to blow on incipient insanity.

The pioneering physicians treating mental illness as a physical complaint relied on the central doctrine of the four humours; all mental imbalance was traceable to some sort of disturbance in the humoural force. The Greeks, having looked at the symptoms, declared that madness divided into two types: melancholia, characterised by depression and withdrawal; and mania, which covered the more aggressive and violent forms of illness. Melancholy was caused by too much black bile; mania was the result of excessive yellow bile. Treatments split into two main camps. One was more gentle than the other and involved bleeding and purging to get rid of the overabundant humour, mixed with rest, massage, exercise and alternating hot and cold baths. Hellebore was the favoured purgative for melancholics, although medical debate raged over whether patients should eat before being forced to expel all into the chamber pot again. Some surgeons, however, favoured more violent methods. Restraints, endless fasting, darkened rooms, dunking in icy water, whipping and bleeding on a heroic scale were all tried.

The Romans adopted the ideas of the Greeks whole-heartedly. In addition to the generally pleasant treatments that existed in Greek medical practice, they built swings and cradles for mentally ill people to sit in, believing that the rocking would soothe the agitated brain. In the second century AD, Celsus, the Roman physician, followed the harsher path, and treated people with violent remedies designed to literally shock them from one mental state to another. Strong emetics and purges, with excessive bleeding and beatings, were followed with large doses of opium to knock out the sufferer. He also recommended shaving the heads of patients and rubbing it with oils, a practice that continued until as recently as the nineteenth century. Other doctors differed. Soranus thought it best not to interfere with the head at all, as this would excite the instability, and instead favoured talking, play-acting and other talking cures, which we would probably recognise today. He believed the root cause of madness was too much wine or too avid a pursuit of gold and fame.

Middle Ages Madness

The Middle Ages was a bad time to be mentally ill in Europe. The generally benign treatments of the Greeks and the Romans were long gone, their texts stolen from the great libraries, or simply forgotten. Instead the influence of the Church grew, and the view of mental illness changed. No longer was insanity the product of imbalanced humours or even various malign spirits. Satan's scheming was at the root of it, and wit-sickness and lunacy were the hallmarks of his activities.

This meant treatment for mental illness was in the hands of the religious and legal professionals of the day; monks, exorcising priests, inquisitors and judges. They would decide the causes, symptoms and treatments for the mentally ill, and they weren't usually pleasant. Mad people were generally allowed to roam free unless they were dangerous, but were often jeered at and persecuted, and sometimes even assaulted and killed. Unsurprisingly a great many mad people very sanely decided leave their homes and took to living in the woods outside the villages, where they could enjoy their unconventional lifestyle undisturbed. The only real danger was if they became deluded, and hastened back into town to tell everyone about some divine visitation they had received. A lynching as a heretic or blasphemer might soon follow.

Mad men, women and children who were submitted for cure invariably found themselves undergoing an exorcism. This cure was prescribed for most types of madness, although there was some recognition that too much drink, old age and a bang on the head could all upset mental balance.

Healing by exorcism was usually practised by the clergy, who were always on the lookout for telltale symptoms of demonic possession: vomiting when taking the Eucharist; aversion to churches; speaking in a strange voice, or telling of events of which they could have no knowledge; loss of appetite; and feeling great weakness. The ceremony of exorcism itself involved the priest approaching the afflicted, who was often pinned or tied down to prevent escape or violence, with a crucifix, which he pressed in the forehead of the 'patient'. Smouldering livers and brains of fish were used to fumigate the patient of demons and prayers were said to force the inhabiting spirit to flee. Beating, whipping and dunking in icy water were also sometimes added, the belief being that it was as well to make the body as inhospitable a place as possible to encourage the demons out. One old English remedy from about 1100 recommended, 'In case a man be lunatic, take the skin of a mere-swine, or porpoise, work it into a whip. Swinge the man therewith, soon he will be well. Amen.' Simple.

The Church, while busy being rotten to the insane, also had their own version of 'good madness', exhibited in the holy ecstasies of saints and visionaries.

ALL IN THE MIND

There were other remedies for mental illness too, which didn't involve getting the priest round. An old Anglo-Saxon remedy was to pound together herbs and roots with ale and holy water. The whole lot was to be left overnight and then drunk the next day from a church bell. Byzantine doctors of the tenth century recommended a course of treatment that lasted two years and required many potions, each successively more bizarre than the last. A patient might have to one day consume the cloak of a recently killed gladiator, following it the next day with the testicles of a young cock washed down with milk; after that the excrement of a dog starved for a week was next on a prescription, which, if it didn't cure the patient, would certainly do nothing for his digestion.

Children who suffered from epilepsy, considered a form of spiritually induced madness, could be cured by eating the brain of a mountain goat, drawn through a golden ring, before they had tasted milk, according to D.H. Tuke's 1882 investigation into ancient British mental health treatments. A side effect meant it could also cure them of seeing apparitions, although it was more likely to permanently cure them of an appetite for offal.

Another remedy for people troubled with hallucinations was wolf's flesh, to be eaten 'well sodden', although sodden with what isn't specified. Anglo-Saxon leech books claimed idiocy could be cured by drinking ale mixed with cassia and

Young men suffering from epilepsy could find themselves castrated to be cured. Some doctors believed that masturbation and sexual excess were the main cause of fits, and so took drastic action to remove the cause and effect of the disorder.

Walnuts, because of their shape, were known as 'brain nuts' and considered good for depression and mental fatigue.

lupins, bishopwort, alexander, fieldmore and holy water. As a bonus cure the leech-doctor generously added the following free advice: 'Against a woman's chatter: taste at night fasting a root of radish, that day the chatter cannot harm thee.'

One shock cure from the Isle of Skye recommended laying the patient, face upwards, on an anvil while the blacksmith took up his heaviest hammer and proceeded to smash it down towards the hapless victim's forehead. At the last possible moment he would feint away, and the blow would pass by harmlessly. The patient, having been so terrified, would be instantly cured.

Shaking was also a recognised cure for most mental illness. The practitioner would take their patient and shake them violently until they would 'snap out of it'. As a remedy it was both cheap and easy to administer. Trepanning was still practised, and a special subset of quacks sprung up in the 1500s, called 'stone doctors'. Discovering someone troubled with mental illness, they would perform an operation, cutting into the patient's scalp and then quickly dropping a stone they had palmed into a basin with a great clank, claiming they had whipped out the physical cause of the problem. This was not a new idea, with the Persian physician Rhazes criticising this practice around 900AD: 'Some wonder doctors claim that they can heal the sickness, they make a cross-shaped opening at the back of the head, and pretend to take something out which they had been holding in their hand . . .'

Because the Devil was the chief cause of mental illness,

extra precautions had to be taken when going abroad after dark, when Satan and his cohorts went about their fiendish work. Prevention was infinitely better than cure if you could get hold of the necessary medicines, which in the case of some remedies could have presented some problems. For example, one twelfth-century English prophylactic against evil advised, 'seek in the maw of young swallows for some little stones and mind that they touch neither earth nor water nor other stones; look out three of them; put them on the man thou wilt, him who hath the need.' Running around a meadow trying to catch young swallows to examine the contents of their beaks was all very well, although you ran the risk of the village idiot moving above you in the social order.

Evil night callers, in league with the Devil, could visit you in your own home and stir up mental turmoil, so it was always just as well to have some efficacious magical salve about just in case they dropped by unannounced. To concoct this one first had to get a few friends round to help gather some choice herbs and shrubs. Once the wormwood, bishopswort, lupin and various other plants were assembled, into a big pot they went, which was then shoved under an altar while your friends joined you in singing nine holy masses, before boiling up the whole lot in sheep's grease and 'much holy salt'. The resultant sludge could then be smeared into the eyes of anyone who had night visitations from evil spirits, it being a certain cure for such cases.

Boneshakers

Shrines and relics were also going great guns at this time, with pilgrimages the pinnacle of many people's lives. Chaucer had written the first road novel, and all over the place people hitched up their feeble or insane relatives and friends and set of in a twitching, limping caravan for a few weeks of relic fondling. These relics, be they bones of dead saints, bits of wood purporting to be from the original cross, or even just the toenail clippings of some holy personage, were considered by most to possess miraculous curative powers. Hawked around the pilgrimages by an assortment of priests and chancers, there were so many shards of supposedly saintly bones around that it would have been possible to reconstruct 12,000 disciples, let alone the original twelve. Nonetheless, faith healing became perhaps the best established form of mental health treatment in the Middle Ages, and special shrines were established to which people travelled from all over Europe. The most famous was that of St Dymphna in Gheel, a town in Belgium still famed for its treatment of the insane. Dymphna was an Irish princess who fled her lunatic father, maddened with incestuous lust for his daughter. Pursuing her, he caught up with her in Gheel where she was buried after he had, in his frenzy, lopped off her head. Miracles began occurring at the site soon after and she was canonised in 1247.

Everyone's Gone Mad

From the thirteenth to the seventeenth century, outbreaks of what appeared to be mass lunacy gripped entire towns and villages. People would be suddenly seized with a compulsion to leap around and dance orgiastically until they collapsed from exhaustion, writhing and twitching. What caused this is open to debate. An outpouring of suppressed sexuality and aggressive instincts? A physical or degenerative condition? Something in the water?

The phenomenon was reported from all over Europe, and

ALL IN THE MIND

It has been suggested that ergot, a mould that thrives in damp conditions and grows on rye used in breadmaking, caused mass hallucinations in people who unknowingly consumed it. However, outbreaks of dance manias occurred at all times of the year, not just at harvest or during wet periods.

became known as the 'dance manias'. Monk and scholar Giraldus Cambrensis witnessed one outbreak in Wales: 'Men and women could be seen in the church singing and dancing. Suddenly they would fall down quite motionless, and then suddenly leap up again like lunatics . . .One man appeared to have a ploughshare in his hands, another urged forward his [imaginary] oxen with his whip.' Dance manias didn't require any musical accompaniment. When bemused onlookers asked what they were doing, the participants replied that they were dancing with devils in a river of blood. Others claimed they had seen the gates of hell open wide beneath their feet. It was assumed that this dancing mania was a special mass lunacy brought on by demon-possession, and exorcisms and religious rites were performed to try to halt the outbreaks.

In the Middle Ages, the madman was generally an undesirable citizen and so, just before the beginning of the Renaissance, instead of driving them out of town, the insane were put on boats and sent out to sea, the original 'ship of fools'. There they would bob about until they drifted into a harbour, whereupon all the locals would come and have a good laugh at them. It may not be as cruel as it sounds, as people believed that the sea and water in general were good for lunacy and so may have thought they were doing the right thing.

Related to these mass outbreaks of lunacy was the Monty Python-esque Brotherhood of Flagellants who roamed Europe at around the same time. Shaven-headed and dressed in long white robes with a red cross on the front, like medieval England football supporters, they roamed across the continent whipping themselves with long leather lashes fitted with iron prongs. This flagellation was, they announced, the only road to salvation, and they would beat themselves until the blood ran down. The Church took a dim view of all this, being the sole appointed agents for salvation-related products, and the popes condemned the Brotherhood's masochistic excesses. However, they only succeeded in driving the movement underground, which would periodically re-emerge during outbreaks of plague and pestilence, seeking new converts as they toured.

The Witch Report

Once Joan of Arc went up in flames for being a witch in 1431, the writing was on the wall for anyone who was suspected of being demon-possessed or in contact with dark forces. If, in the Middle Ages, lunatics had been suspected of insanity via possession and in need of exorcism to be cured, then the Renaissance period marked a turn for the worse for any unfortunate sufferers. Progressively, those suspected of possession weren't just branded lunatics and raving fools, but dangerous heretics in league with the Devil. This new dogma brought a new treatment: from now on, perfidious lunatics wouldn't be cured by exorcisms or sprinklings of holy water. Instead the Devil would be driven out of his hosts by burning. As a medical treatment for insanity, this was an example of the cure being infinitely worse than the disease, but the natural antidote to this type of thinking, analytical medicine, although not in full retreat, was certainly keeping a lower profile at this time. A few doctors did venture to suggest that insanity was a disease with physical, not spiritual, origins, but most, even if they did harbour doubts, kept their heads down. After all, such was the temper of the times that to openly question the prevalent doctrine could quickly see you accused of heresy too.

This gradual change from viewing mad people – especially women – as dangerous and malevolent witches rather than simple lunatics took place against a background of medical ambivalence about mental illness. Mr Caxton's press meant the writings of the Greeks and Romans with their emphasis on physical cures were becoming available again, but the old superstitions persisted.

Sometimes the two got mixed up as in the example of Guy de Chauliac, a fourteenth-century physician who believed that trepanation was highly therapeutic for the insane, but should on no account be undertaken under a full moon, as the Devil was likely to leap into any freshly bored hole. Others around the same time claimed that insanity was brought about by over-warm humours, which seemed classical Greek diagnosis. But, they added, the hot bile attracted the Devil who liked to inhabit a warm nest, and that was the real cause of the problem.

By the mid-fifteenth century, the distinction between a mentally ill person and a heretic had blurred sufficiently to

To cure mental illness, sufferers would be bound to holy crosses, often overnight. This would scare the demons out of them, and by morning they would be sane once again.

ensure that anyone who was afflicted with insanity could be charged with witchcraft. A handbook published in 1486, commissioned by the Church and written by two Dominican monks, served as a guide to diagnosing witchcraft in the insane. Entitled *Malleus Maleficarum*, it informed the reader how to identify, examine and sentence a witch. Witch courts were convened and the accused brought before them to be cross-questioned and medically examined for marks of the Devil. The courts insisted on confession, and, sadly, the confused and often bewildered mentally ill victims brought before them would agree that they were witches, without the faintest understanding of what they were really doing.

Stories were often bizarre, as in the case of a young woman, Sara Williams, who was examined for witchcraft in 1585. Possession had taken place when a cat jumped out of a bush at her when she was a girl; she claimed that she had

According to *Malleus Maleficarum*, the Devil was believed to leave marks on the skin of his accomplices, often in secret or hidden places. To identify these marks, people who were accused of witchcraft had their bodies shaved and appeared before the courts naked, where a thorough examination was carried out. Anything like a mole or a birthmark could be deemed a Devil's mark, and evidence enough of diabolic activity. If no mark could be found, then the accused would be pricked with needles, as the Devil in his cunning may have left an invisible mark. However, the skilled witchfinder would still be able to find this spot as it would be insensitive to pain even when stabbed. It is known today that people suffering with hysterical mental conditions often have areas of 'dead' skin and this test would have been horribly accurate for people with this form of illness.

also swallowed a green and black dog, which had 'burnt her heart'. The trial reported that she was highly productive of devils; sometimes during fits she managed to produce a quartet who sang rounds together 'in measure and sweet cadence'. Luckily for her she was deemed curable and was treated through fumigation with singed fish guts, escaping full-scale burning. For those who wouldn't confess, or had enough of their wits about them to realise what was going on, agonising tortures were devised to get them to talk. Devices like the Witch's Bridle were commonly applied – an iron collar with a metal tongue, which went into the mouth and had spikes which pierced the palate, tongue and soft inner cheek. The Spanish Boot was another favourite, a wooden shoe that could be screwed tighter and tighter, crushing the bones in the foot.

Witch trials took place all over Europe, and the mentally ill population of many towns and villages were put on trail for communing with the Devil. Soon the definition of madness was widened to include any symptoms of involuntary non-conformity. People denounced their neighbours as witches for harmless eccentric behaviour, nervous tics and even muttering to themselves. Unscrupulous men used the climate of fear to get rid of nagging wives or difficult neighbours. God-fearing men and women blamed everyday illnesses on bewitchment, and cast about for someone to blame.

Some doctors did voice their opposition to the obsession with witchcraft. Paracelsus took a stand, claiming that 'nature is the sole origin of diseases' (he also believed that the brain had an exterior stomach, which resided in the upper part of the nose). Another medical student and scholar, Johann Weyer, went further and published his work

De Praestigiis Daemonum (On Witchcraft) in 1563 where he denounced the persecution of sick people and instead recommended their torturers be punished instead (the book was listed as prohibited by the Catholic Church until the twentieth century). Unscrupulous quacks flourished, using the climate of fear and suspicion to convince trembling patients that their ailments were the result of malign influences. One story told how in a tavern in 1567 a man approached a quack who had recently cured his master of a stammer. The man was sick, and wanted to obtain the services of this 'physician' to make him well again. After a quick examination, the illness, pronounced the quack, was of demonic origins. For an exorbitant fee he could guarantee a cure, but if his recommendations were not followed then this terrible illness would spread throughout the man's family, and even into his cattle. Returning to the man's home, he confined him to his bedchamber while he embarked upon elaborate rituals, filled with mumbo-jumbo designed to impress and frighten the patient's young daughter. Muttering incantations over an old book, he arranged knives in the shape of the cross and asked her to participate in placing them in a 'charmed' circle he had constructed. Forcing a morsel of food on her (she was to later claim it was ice-cold as if from the Devil himself), the young woman became disturbed and confused and felt as if she were losing control of her senses. The quack then told her to bare her breasts and loosen her girdle, and proceeded to have sex with her. The girl was reluctant to cooperate, but the 'doctor' assured her that if she did not her father was sure to die, and she herself would fall ill with the same malady. Flesh to flesh contact was, he insisted, medically necessary. This 'treatment' was repeated the next day, while the father was meanwhile

Agnes Sampson was tried for witchcraft in 1590 for attempting to cure a Robert Carr. Using spells she took his disease upon herself, and, after a painful night, in the morning tried to transfer it to her cat. Unfortunately her aim was off and she instead transferred the disease to a local man, Alex Douglas, who promptly died.

dosed with such large draughts of poison that he was confined to bed in great agony. Eventually he summoned his daughter to his bedchamber to find out how the good doctor was progressing with his treatment. Noticing her shame and embarrassment, he wheedled the whole story out of her. The quack fled, and, duplicitous to the end, was last reported living a happy, if full, life. 'Everyone in town knows that, old as he is, he has taken a second wife, even though the first is still living,' reported his biographer.

Other medical impostors got in on the act too. On young man, suffering from a swollen belly, was convinced by a doctor in Cleves that he was bewitched and was nursing in his belly a venerable but malicious viper with two red rings around its neck, accompanied by a couple of younger serpents. This was so implausible even in those days that the doctor was watched closely to make sure that he didn't slip some dead snakes into the chamber pot, which was frequently filled from the violent purges he employed in his treatment. In desperation he invented a story that the sick boy would experience birth pangs, and he, the doctor, would need to put his hands on the patient's private parts beneath the bedclothes to deliver the snakes. The mother, who had been forewarned about such quackish tricks, refused to allow this, and so the doctor failed, fleeing before the patient died.

English Disease

As the preoccupation with witchcraft died out, rational analysis was once again applied to ideas about mental illness, and new ideas forged. Learned men applied themselves to the problems and causes of mental illness, and new conclusions were drawn. One of these was that mental instability, particularly the variety known as melancholy, was especially prevalent amongst Englishmen. The ball was set rolling by the scholar and melancholic Robert Burton. His morose masterwork *The Anatomy of Melancholy,* which was published first in 1621, remained popular until the late nineteenth century, and was reprinted many times. The book examined the causes of melancholy, its symptoms, and methods for escaping its grip. Chapters with cheery titles such as, 'An Heape of other accidents causing melancholy. Death of Friends, losses etc.' and 'A digression of the misery of schollars' detailed the complaints that attended the unhappy melancholic. Students, opined Burton, were miserable because the time they spent in academic contemplation 'dries the braine, and extinguisheth naturall heat'. Further-more, scholars lacked any social graces: 'they cannot ride an horse, which every Clowne can doe; salute and court a Gentlewoman, carve at table . . . which every common swasher can doe'. Their misery was compounded by being poor, taking no exercise and suffering long periods of solitude. Other types of depression categorised by the glum but prolific Burton were, in no particular order: Head melancholy; Terrors and afrights; Digression of spirits; and Windie Melancholy.

Cures listed certainly didn't hold out the promise of easy happiness in a pill that we expect today. But then a lot of the

Redness and blushing were thought to afflict melancholy and depressed people. Washing the face with hare's blood at night, and applying fresh cheese curds when the redness took hold were two approved seventeenth-century remedies.

symptoms described by doctors at the time are not the familiar modern associations with melancholy or depression: 'withered', 'much troubled with winde', 'flaggy beardes', 'singing of the eares' and 'wrinckled' were all notable indicators of English Disease.

Some relief could be obtained through medicines. Although Burton was sceptical about doctors – 'Physitians kill as many as they save, & who can tell . . . how many murders they make in a yeare' – he was wise enough to make sure he didn't alienate the medical profession. 'I am well perswaded of Physick,' he wrote, in case one day, 'some Physitian should mistake me, & deny me Physick when I am sick.' It's difficult not to share his scepticism. One rare cure he described was for 'dotage, head melancholie, and such diseases of the braine' and called for a ram's head (one that had never 'meddled with an Ewe'), cut off with one blow and the horns removed and the whole thing 'skinne and wooll together' boiled until soft. The brain was removed, spices sprinkled on it, and then cooked up on hot coals. This was fed to the patient for three days, who had to fast in between

An old Arabic remedy recommended for melancholy, fears and palpitations: the flesh of a hawk flavoured with cloves, and white wine instead of water.

these 'meals'. Another remedy called for the lungs of a ram 'applied hot to the forepart of the head', or if no rams were available, a young lamb split along the spine. Shepherds had to be especially watchful of their flocks when melancholic young men were around.

Bezoars (calcified stones from the stomachs of ruminants) taken in water of ox-tongue were thought to be useful in treating depressives, and Burton noted that the Turks used a drink called coffa, 'of a berry as blacke as soot, and as bitter', consumed in coffa houses and which seemed to help digestion and 'procureth alacrity' (a desirable quality against melancholy).

The English susceptibility to melancholy was therefore well known, and even celebrated. Also known as spleen or hypochondriasis, it was said to be a sign of unusual gifts or sensibility in a person. Unsurprisingly, this was an affliction found only amongst the refined and socially respectable classes, the depressed unwashed poor being merely lunatics worthy only of incarceration. 'English malady' was said to be caused by the moist air, variable weather, over-rich diet and overpopulation of the British Isles, and displayed itself as a melancholic depression in sufferers. Other symptoms included runny nose, fever and stomach aches.

Against this background came a change in the way that mental illness, and particularly melancholy, was treated. Out went the harsh physical treatments of old, and in came new therapies, which tried gentle persuasion in a family-like setting. One cure, which was perhaps the most appropriate for the mentally weak English, was that devised by William Tuke. A Quaker, Tuke opened an asylum in York in about 1792, which tried to treat its inmates with some kindness and respect, and a key therapy was that of tea. Each afternoon the patients would take tea in a civilised way, the idea being that this ceremony would teach them how to behave and control their behaviour in a social environment. No finer confirmation of sanity was there than an Englishman able to enjoy a cup of tea in a civilised manner. Other contemporary treatments involved warm baths (often for hours on end), overfeeding (to promote healing sleep) and exercise.

No Hiding Place

The first lunatic asylum was opened in 1247 in London. The Priory of St Mary of Bethlehem was initially set up as a monastery, but it soon began functioning as a hospital accommodating the mentally sick. By the end of the fourteenth century Bedlam was established, a word that became synonymous with the madhouse, uproar and mental chaos. The image of the hospital as a dungeon, packed with howling, raving lunatics captured the popular imagination. Hogarth used it as the final scene of *A Rake's Progress*, the anti-hero Tom Rakehell finishing up in Bedlam as a reward for his dissolute life.

Being thrown into Bedlam (or into any mental hospital in Europe) between the thirteenth and eighteenth centuries was something to be feared. Treatments were brutal, and there was little prospect of cure for any of the inmates. Control and restraint were the order of the day, the main mission being to keep out of the sight of society insane undesirables. Patients were chained up, and left naked in cells for years on end and beatings were frequent and vicious. Lunatics were believed to have lost their reason, the only thing to set humans apart from animals. Without this they were little more than beasts,

ALL IN THE MIND

and it was thought that they were both insensible as well as for the most part incurable. Those patients singled out for treatment were likely to suffer in the name of medicine. Beating was considered a cure for some cases, a view subscribed to by Thomas More in 1553, who reported a man 'put up in bedelem, and afterwarde by betyinge and correccyon gathered hys remembraunce to hym'. Some medicines were also available, but didn't go down well with patients: 'Hellish Physick, Quack down my throat does pour,' moaned one inmate in 1670. Generally, purging, vomits, bleeding and bathing were the order of the day, although there were exceptions to this routine.

Fear was a well-known cure for mental illness, and most asylum doctors agreed that it was a useful remedy. In the United States Benjamin Rush, a leading medical figure, thought terror a very efficient tool, and wasn't averse to unexpectedly dunking his asylum patients into ice-cold water through trapdoors to frighten them, once even threatening to kill a woman to provide a therapeutic jolt to her system. He was the inventor of the tranquillising chair in which inmates were held utterly immobile with a wooden box strapped to their head blocking off sight and sound. But he was most proud of his Gyrator, a device in which the patient was strapped to a board or chair, and the whole thing was spun around as fast as possible, the theory being that blood would rush to the head and relieve the congested brain. Other asylums used devices like the Utica Crib, a small cage like a

More people are admitted to mental hospitals in the summer than at any other time of the year.

Water shock cures. Benjamin Rush wasn't the first person to use the shock of being plunged into icy water as a cure for madness. For centuries people had been trying this method of cure, with a variety of cunning ruses. Sometimes unsuspecting patients were sat on a stool and an icy jet of water was suddenly directed on to their anus. Others were lured into boats designed to break up when halfway across a lake. Some found themselves walking over bridges which would collapse when halfway across, dropping them into the icy streams below.

coffin in which patients were put for hours on end, so constricted that they could not even turn their heads.

'Now I guess I'll have to tell 'em / That I've got no cerebellum' – The Ramones

The lunatic asylums provided the testing grounds for many new therapies. One of these is electro convulsive therapy, or ECT, which, although identified with twentieth-century medicine (and Jack Nicholson's fried brains in *One Flew Over the Cuckoo's Nest*), was first used in 47 AD when Scribonius Largus employed an electric eel to treat the headaches of the Roman emperor. The same technique was used by the Jesuit missionaries to Abyssinia in the sixteenth century, who would apply an electric catfish to drive out the tormenting devils of the mentally ill. Probably the first recorded ECT treatment using an electricity generating machine was that carried out by French doctor J-B. LeRoy in 1755. John Wesley, evangelist and part-time medical man, wrote in 1760 that electricity was 'the general and rarely failing Remedy in nervous cases of every kind' and was the proud possessor of his own electrical machine. Bedlam got its first electric therapy instrument in 1796 (although neither patients nor doctors thought much of it). The idea that electrical current was generally invigorating and beneficial to health was widespread and had many followers, but it wasn't until the twentieth century that ECT really came into its own. Behind its popularity was the idea that applying an electric current to the head of a mentally ill person would shock their system back into a normal pattern, an idea no more sophisticated than the Middle Ages idea of dousing someone unexpectedly with icy water to cure them. Nonetheless ECT therapy, perhaps because of its veneer of technological sophistication, survived and gained ground, peaking in its use in the 1940s and 1950s. Thousands of people were given shocks, from three-year-old children to ninety-six-year-old spinsters. Sometimes the jolts given were so severe, bones would snap and teeth smash as the patient convulsed on the table, and many patients were treated against their will. Results varied; some people, especially those with depression, responded well. Others experienced no benefit, and were damaged by the treatment. By the 1970s the practice of administering ECT was being challenged by ex-patients and doctors and it gradually fell from favour, although it is still used in some hospitals today.

The Unkindest Cut

Another controversial treatment was psychosurgery, or to the layman, lobotomy. Although trepanning and other outbreaks of head-sawing had taken place through history, it was during the late nineteenth and early twentieth century that speculation began about tinkering with the brain to modify (and possibly cure) the behaviour of mad people.

The initial interest in tampering with the brain to change behaviour was triggered by an accident that befell a railway worker, Phineas Gage, in 1848. An explosion drove a length of pipe through his forehead and into his brain. Despite losing lots of blood, Phineas was up and about almost immediately and made a full recovery. However, his friends soon noticed that his personality was much changed. Instead of being his usual agreeable self he had turned into a violent and angry character, prone to rages and black moods (understandable perhaps, with a lump of pipe sticking out of his head). Childlike in his intellect and given to sudden bursts of ripe language, he eventually went on to tour as a sideshow attraction with P.T. Barnum, and crowds came to gawp at the man who walked around with a piece of plumbing protruding from his brain. His case intrigued doctors and they speculated whether the injury to the brain was responsible for Phineas's changed behaviour. At the same time doctors started to notice that patients with brain tumours that destroyed areas of the brain also experienced personality changes, and after considering these and other facts, a Dr Egas Moniz was persuaded to take up his scalpel in 1935 and perform the first human lobotomy (before he carried out this operation he had experimented on cadavers, ferrying their severed heads around Lisbon in his chauffeur-driven limousine). Practising his technique before operating on a live patient by jabbing his fountain pen repeatedly into a practice brain he had acquired, the surgical procedure was carried out on a sixty-three-year-old woman who had been diagnosed as an involuntary melancholic with paranoia. The operation was deemed a success, Moniz reporting that the woman appeared calm and rational after a few days of recovery.

Effectively a method of destroying bits of the brain, this

The human brain on average weighs 2–3lb and smells of strong blue cheese.

new technique was considered a huge breakthrough in the treatment of mental illness, gained world-wide fame, and was taken up by two American doctors, Freeman and Watts. Over the years they developed their own brand of lobotomy (involving a sharp point and a hammer), which they even practised on patients in their offices. The spike, usually an ice pick, would be driven into the brain with a hammer through the eye socket, then the handle levered upwards, cracking the bones around the eye and cutting deep into the brain tissue. Violent, and unproven, it was nonetheless an easy operation to do and didn't even require a hospital stay. Freeman was one day disturbed operating in his office, a patient slumped over his desk with an ice pick sticking out from above one eye.

With a robust attitude towards the brain, Freeman became an increasingly enthusiastic advocate for lobotomy, performing them at the drop of the hat, in one case lobotomising an unconscious man in his motel room. He had a less than clinical attitude towards other medical disciplines though, for example instructing a colleague to forget about 'all that germ crap' when carrying out brain surgery. Between 1949 and 1952 lobotomies were at their peak, with 5,000 per year being carried out in the USA. Yet by the mid-1950s the practice had fallen from favour and psychosurgery began to decline. In part this was due to the indiscriminate selection of patients who were often chosen not for their symptoms but their availability, but was mainly because of the post-operative effects. After having their skulls cracked and shafts of brain minced and removed like the core out of an apple,

QUACK MAGIC

Responsible for at least five deaths, 'Dr Jones' was in fact a former mental patient who bluffed his way into the Chicago practice of a holidaying doctor. He was finally exposed by a nurse in whom he had become romantically interested. Her suspicions were aroused when on making his rounds he mispronounced medical terms and prescribed the wrong medicines. After having his advances rebuffed, Dr Jones tried to choke the nurse, which moved her to enquire about his suitability to practice medicine. She discovered he was not in fact the celebrated graduate of Northwestern University he claimed to be. When the police came to arrest him they found that his black doctor's bag contained a vast quantity of morphine and a gun.

many patients became not only calm and docile as intended, but also mentally dulled and indifferent to their surroundings and environment. Some ended up having to wear nappies and be cared for like small children, and even where some patients managed to return to some semblance of normal life, the symptoms that led them to be lobotomised in the first place often returned. Although some doctors argued that it was better for people who suffered from mental illness to have a dulled mind rather than a disordered one, other people vehemently opposed this view, some even drawing parallels with Nazi medical experimentation. It is estimated that between 1945 and 1960, over 70,000 lobotomies were carried out in the US and Britain alone.

Talking Crazy and Other Cures

The twentieth century has seen a variety of cures for madness come and go, some which have caught on and others that have gone out of fashion. Cocaine addict and cake-fancier Sigmund Freud effectively started the 'talking cure' where patients discussed, explored and subsequently resolved their neuroses with his theories of the repressed unconscious. Different varieties of this exist – there is Freudian analysis, Jungian analysis, family therapy, group sessions – but they all share a belief that the remedy to a mental problem can be 'talked out'. These cures are legitimate and mainstream, preferable by far to having the front of your brain teased out with a knitting needle as a cure for depression. But there exists a far wilder shore of modern psychiatric treatment, occupying the uneven territory between the physical cures of the Middle Ages and the talking cures we know today.

Past-life therapy is a well-known psychiatric treatment firmly associated with quackism. Described by the head of the American Psychiatric Association as 'charlatanism at its finest', the general idea is that the patient is 'regressed' by the therapist using hypnotherapy so that they can relive their past lives. By doing this they will discover the past traumas and personality traits from their earlier incarnations that are still bombarding their current subconscious. On coming out of their trance these discoveries will enable them to resolve their issues and attain better mental health. Two things are immediately noticeable about these regressions. One is social climbing. Where are all the midden-heap attendants and swineherds from the past? Everyone who revisits their former lives is invariably of royal blood or some kind of favoured noble, lording it over the rabble. The other is that (and it's hard to separate it from the first point) it has been proved people will remember things that never happened, otherwise known as false memory syndrome. Scientific studies have shown that past-life reports are mainly influenced by the patient's suggestibility and proneness to fantasise. If they were told that previous incarnations are often of a different sex and culture, then this is what they generally incorporated into their past-life descriptions. This may seem harmless enough, but over the last fifteen years, hundreds of ill-trained quacks, often calling themselves 'traumatists', have set themselves up in business with disastrous results. Encouraging patients to 'remember' past childhood traumas, incest, rapes and alien abductions has led to prosecutions for events that never took place, and families breaking apart. In 1993, recognising the problem, a group of doctors set up a false memory foundation to deal with the problems of adults who mistakenly believed they were the victims of childhood abuse. Within twelve months they had received over 4,000 calls from families who had been attacked by their offspring, accusing them of deeds that hadn't taken place.

Substitute the word 'quack' for 'therapist' and suddenly some of these treatments seem a lot closer to the medicine show days of old. If the mind is the new medical frontier, there are plenty of cowboys still riding the range. Worried and anxious about your relationship with your children, for example? A course of rebirthing treatment will resolve the

Past-life mania swept the nation in the 1950s. Under hypnosis, a woman from Ireland began telling tales from the nineteenth century, when she had apparently been a maid called Bridey Murphy. Her hypnotists wrote a best-selling book about the case, which was later revealed as a fraud. 'Bridey' had in fact just been recounting tales told to her by her nanny.

problems, or at least this was what one patient was told when she visited a 'therapist'. To resolve her issues, claimed the quack, the patient would have to re-experience her own birth and development, giving her a second chance to 'grow up right'. The sessions consisted of being rolled in a carpet, which the patients had to wriggle out of, just as they squirmed out of the birth canal years ago. Hungry from the birthing, patients would be fed either with a bottle or set to suckle at the therapist's breast. They would, of course, be wearing nappies throughout, and would be encouraged to soil themselves with abandon. Rebirthing therapy or 'corrective parenting' is fairly widespread, no doubt encouraged by the tendency of everybody to blame their parents for their problems. Not only is it practised in America, but in England as well. A damning report by a Birmingham newspaper uncovered a rebirthing centre where patients were tied by pieces of rope to their therapists and had to crawl round on the floor like babies.

If rebirthing isn't appropriate, then someone, somewhere, will have developed a suitable cure. Ever-inventive quacks have latched on to enough bizarre theories to ensure that there is a profitable treatment available for the most picky customers: Angel therapy (contacting and chatting with

A leading light in the rebirthing world claims she tried to communicate with her mother from inside the womb, informing her that she wanted to be born at home. She also tried to communicate with her mother's doctors, apparently. Her mother heard her, she says, and she was born in a home delivery. Sadly though, birth took place on the kitchen table, which has resulted in her having a lifelong food neurosis.

angels to resolve problems, facilitated by an experienced 'therapist'); Orgone therapy (collecting invisible 'life force' by sitting in a wooden box, available by mail order); White Goddess healing (invocations, via an expert, to a white female deity who can bestow mental calmness); Soul work (awakening latent pieces of DNA to enable intuitive self-healing); and Drumming (banging the path to better health by hitting a drum) are just a few treatments available. Some modern therapies don't even bother to hide the fact that they're just the same old remedies recycled. For Hypnotism read Mesmerism. Devotees of 'shamanic counselling' seem to not mind that this went out with communicating with the spirits and sabre-toothed tigers.

The Truth Is Out There

Some of the therapies are so strange that it is bemusing that anyone actually crosses the therapist's doorstep. Firmly in this camp is alien abduction therapy, whose proponents claim that the mental problems people suffer are the result of aliens whisking them off for a bout of experimentation before dumping their probed bodies back on to earth. These extraterrestrial one-night stands are responsible for, amongst other conditions, depression, psychosis and an increased appetite for conspiracy theories. Usually 'discovered' using hypnosis, one helpful therapist offers in her book a method for DIY abduction detection. 'You can discover your own close encounters,' she enthuses. Take a piece of string with a small weight on the end and learn to 'will' the pendulum to swing in different directions; back and forth for 'yes' and side to side for 'no'. Once this has been mastered, the reader should work though fifty set questions, such as: Have I ever seen a UFO? Have I received telepathic messages from ETs? and Am I a human-alien hybrid? Each one should be answered by a swing of the pendulum. At the end of it all, a definitive answer on the question of whether or not your life was in fact just a bad episode of *The X-Files* would emerge. There are even checklists of symptoms and indicators of alien abduction, which include:

Memory of little grey men in the bedroom;
Dreams of intrusive medical procedures;
Waking up with a sense of dread;
Other family members being abducted;
Fear of night time, hospitals, flying, elevators, animals, insects, sex, loneliness, the dark, exposed windows;
Rashes, nosebleeds, cuts, sinus pain, rectal bleeding;
Difficult pregnancy; stomach and bowel complaints.

What this list reveals is that not only are most of us likely to know someone with at least one of these complaints, but that haemorrhoids are caused by aliens as well. Pile sufferers can now speculate freely on the whether there is intelligent life out there, and if so, what is it doing poking around between their buttocks? ET therapists claim that an average of more than 3,000 close encounters occur every twenty-four hours in the US alone, which if nothing else means that these quacks won't be short of patients for a while.

 Some psychologists have likened the growing spate of abductions in the US to the outbreaks of mass hysteria of the 'dance manias' of the Middle Ages.

Let It All Out

One therapy is the idea of catharsis for relief of mental problems. This is not a new idea. The Ancient Greeks believed in venting feelings by going to the theatre and emoting along with the characters, draining off emotions like pity and fear. Sensibly though, the Greeks tended to leave it at that and no doubt went home with a lighter step to paint some urns and catch up on the latest Aristotle. Modern society, though, is not so enlightened. Cathartic therapies abound, with different schools of thought. Popular in the 1970s was primal scream therapy, one devotee being John Lennon. Through animalistic screaming, patients release the pent-up rage in their elemental core, laying to rest their mental problems. Variations exist, like the Mystic Rose based on the teachings of the guru Bhagwan Shree Rajnesh, where laughing and crying fits are supposed to open the doors to personal healing. Attack therapy revolves around the unfortunate patient being abused and insulted by members of his therapy group and his therapist, the brutal assaults somehow resulting in a cure for whatever mental problems brought them there in the first place. Some therapists even encourage patients to attack each other physically, giving them plastic cudgels to work out their anger on each other. Never ones to miss a trick, cases have been reported where the quack has encouraged two patients to go at each other hammer and tongs, and then sent them a bill the next day for damage to his premises. Cathartic therapy has been demonstrated to actually have the opposite effect to the one it claims, qualifying it for entry into the quack hall of fame. Research has shown that rather than dissipate and release anger, urging people to behave in a hostile and violent manner encourages this type of behaviour.

One woman in the USA who attended scream therapy actually became so enraged that she tried to kill her husband before shooting herself in the head.

Knock Some Sense In

Modern therapy doesn't always have to revolve around talking, screaming, wearing a nappy or hypnosis. Physical cures still have their place, although they are far from accepted mainstream medical practice. Offering fast, magical quick-fixes for mental illness, practitioners can become certified (usually by an institute founded by the inventor of the technique), which adds an aura of professional respectability. Treatments like neural organisation technique (NOT) are so physical that people who have carried them out have been successfully sued for battery. Based on the theories of Carl Ferreri, NOT rests on the premise that breathing causes the bones of the skull to move about. This in turn is responsible for various problems like dyslexia, cerebral palsy and learning difficulties. By manipulating these skull bones the NOT doctor claims he can offer relief from these conditions. Despite the fact that medical textbooks state the bones of the skull are pretty firmly welded together and cannot move about, and that there is no evidence to back up these claims, this hasn't stopped NOT being used on children. One school in California hired Ferreri and associates to practise on the children enrolled there, an episode that resulted in court actions for fraud and malpractice.

Rapid eye movement, or to give it its full name eye movement desensitisation and reprocessing, is a less violent, but still bizarre practice. 'Discovered' by a psychologist in the late 1980s, it essentially promotes the idea that rapid flickering eye movements can be used to reduce anxiety and unpleasant thoughts. Having stumbled upon this medical breakthrough by chance while wandering in the park, the doctor soon launched the procedure on the world with over 14,000 people training (for a fee) to use the technique. Especially useful in treating stress disorders, it has been used to heal people mentally scarred by diverse experiences: rape, molestation, Vietnam combat and natural disasters, apparently. Painless to administer, the therapist swings their fingers like a hypnotist's watch in front of the patient's eyes, while the patient summons up troubling thoughts. As their eyes flicker from side to side following the finger, the trauma they are remembering evaporates. Does it work? No studies exist to show that this technique has any therapeutic value whatsoever.

Whether they're here in ten or twenty years, or will have become as outdated as such medieval practices as whipping for madness (which could quite feasibly be even now the very latest word in contemporary therapy), it is hard to say. History shows that cures spring up, are briefly fashionable, and then discredited, to be supplanted by equally bizarre methods. In the not very distant future, Roman remedies could be back in fashion and concoctions of turtle blood and hellesbore will have replaced regression, chanting and banging drums in the woods.

QUACK ALUMNI

Members of the quack fraternity span the centuries. Some of them are so closely bonded with specific illnesses and treatments that their name has become a synonym for quackish practices – mesmerism for example. But others have happily flitted from one illness to the next, not bound to one condition alone, but instead nobly dedicating themselves to charlatanism and fraud in a whole host of medical spheres. Specialist or generalist, eccentrics or calculating fraudsters, these people provided alternative medicine long before the phrase was even invented.

Early Exports

Namechecked by Chaucer in the Prologue to *The Canterbury Tales*, Gilbert the Englishman was the first English physician

In the Dark Ages physicians were forced to leave a cash sum with the household of their patient. If they died, the family kept the money and didn't have to pay the bill.

to make his name abroad with remedies like this splendid 1230 cure for gout:

Take a frog when neither sun nor moon is shining; cut off its hind legs and wrap them in deer skin; apply the right to the right and the left to the left foot of the gouty person, and without doubt he will be healed.

Claudius of Rome was choked to death by his doctor, who tickled his throat with a feather in an attempt to make him vomit.

Dropping Pills

Joshua 'Spot' Ward was one of the most successful quacks and patent medicine vendors. He made an absolute fortune, and when his will was published in 1762, a year after his death, society was agog at the details. After an introduction in which he generously forgave all his enemies, from the grave he rubbed salt in their wounds by flaunting his wealth in his bequests; £2,000 to his niece, £100 to his coachman and a string of properties to be distributed amongst various legatees.

The medicine that had amassed him this wealth was the famous Pill and Drop. Essentially the same medicine, it didn't matter in which form it was taken. Astute quack that Ward was though, he noticed that some people just couldn't swallow pills and, like drugs manufacturers today, ensured in his patent Drop that there was a liquid product. Before he became a patent medicine manufacturer Ward had been an MP. However, he was removed from his seat when it transpired that he had somehow contrived to be elected without actually obtaining a single vote. He went abroad, returning sixteen years later in 1733 with the recipe for his famous medicines. Ward started intensive advertising of his products, and was helped by testimonies of astonishing cures which his Pill and Drop reportedly effected: one, a young woman, lay at death's door after two months of traditional medical treatment. Bled, purged, blistered and vomited, she was so weakened and emaciated that she couldn't even open and close her eyelids without the help of her nurse. In desperation she was given Ward's medicine. The effects were immediate, if disconcerting; she began to pour sweat and vomit uncontrollably. Remarkably, though, she began to recover. Within days she had dispensed with the services of her nurse and was up and about, walking in the garden and doing needlework (eighteenth-century proof of a woman restored to full health).

However, not all Ward's press was good, as was demonstrated in the case of a Mrs Gilbert who took some of Ward's pills in 1734. After swallowing them she vomited thirty-four times, and purged her bowels twenty-two times (whoever

George Berkeley (1685–1753) the Irish Anglican bishop and philosopher, was an empiric (those, like John Wesley, who regarded themselves as scientists and used remedies in an experimental way, noting their effects and saving them for future use). Berkeley was a keen promoter of Tar Water – literally water mixed with tar, left to stand and drunk off. He believed Tar Water cured smallpox, scurvy, hysteria, plague, 'all diseases of the urinary passage', gout, gangrene and piles. Tar Water fell out fashion, largely due to its inability to effect any of the cures it promised.

collected these statistics showed commendable diligence). All this stomach trouble almost inevitably caused serious problems, and Mrs Gilbert 'miserably died' the next night. This, of course, showed Ward and his medicines in a bad light, and he launched a propaganda counter-offensive. Sworn testimony from Mrs Gilbert's servant Jane revealed in sensational fashion that Mrs Gilbert was a 'gross, fat woman' who was fed up with her constantly griping guts. She had, alleged Jane, taken every remedy available from the apothecary to get rid of her digestive complaint, including the Pill and Drop, which alone had brought her relief. On the evening she had taken the fatal dose, she had washed it down with a fine meal of bacon and greens. Ward was off the hook; all his medicines had printed instructions forbidding both greens and milk to those taking them. Mrs Gilbert had ignored these warnings and had paid the price. Ward defended other similar cases in the same way, either by arguing that patients had contravened his instructions, or were so far gone that no medicine could have saved them anyway.

Ward didn't need to worry about unfavourable press – after all he could count the King of England amongst his supporters. After resetting the dislocated thumb of George II to royal satisfaction, he became a court favourite and was given a Whitehall apartment and permission to drive his coach through St James's Park. This patronage was exceedingly useful to Ward; when the Apothecaries Act was passed in 1748 to put a stop to the unlicensed trade in medicines, a clause was specifically included that exempted him.

Ward wasn't purely concerned with profit, however; he opened hospitals in three London houses to dispense medicine and treatment to the poor, and he often distributed money as well. For a while it was fashionable for socialites of the day to assist in dispensing Ward's Pill and Drop to the needy in his hospitals.

So what was in the Pill and Drop? A recipe from a miscellany published in the late 1700s called for dragon's blood, 'rich mountain wine', and antimony. This last ingredient was the key. Antimony is a chemical that can cause violent sickness and diarrhoea, decay and nephritis (rotting of the intestines) and even bring about death from shock. It isn't used in medicine today, but did enjoy great popularity in the past. Not unknown to most amateur chemists at the time, Ward's medicine was probably no different from other products.

On the Road

One of the physicians of Charles II was a well-known quack. One of his special remedies was a potion called Orvietan, which he insisted was an effective antidote to all poisons. To demonstrate this he encouraged challengers to concoct the vilest poison they could. He would administer it to one of his servants, restoring him with a dose of Orvietan to prove its potency. What he didn't reveal was that he forced the servant to gorge himself on butter beforehand. When the challengers came forward with the poison they had prepared, the poor man's mouth and gullet were so smeared with butter that the poison couldn't be absorbed. Under instruction though, he would drink it down, collapse as if dead and be carted away. The next day he would be paraded by the triumphant quack, no worse off for his ordeal, proof that his poison antidote worked; what had really happened was that once he was out

QUACK MAGIC

> Quacks and mountebanks who toured the country were often accompanied by jesters called 'zanies' or a 'merry Andrew' whose job it was to draw a crowd and entertain them while his master cried up his wares.

of sight he had been fed more butter, which made him vomit up all the poison. Another trick by the same doctor was used to sell his Green Salve, which he claimed could cure any wound. Spectators were treated to the sight of a man appearing to plunge his hands into a bowl of molten lead. He seemed to suffer terrible burns, screaming in agony, and the doctor would immediately spring forward with his Green Salve, which he applied before bandaging up the man's hands. The next day, however, the bandages would be removed in public and the hands revealed to be quite healed. The crowd probably wouldn't have gasped with such amazement if they realised they had been duped; the molten lead was in fact liquid mercury, and quite cold.

A Man of Science

Dr Katterfelto, the self-described 'greatest philosopher in this kingdom', was a London quack who practised 'medicine' from about 1780 until his death in 1799. His speciality was influenza, which he claimed to be able to cure with the help of his magnificent invention, the Solar Microscope. Posing foremost as a man of science, Katterfelto was a sort of scientific conjuror who gave shows involving lectures on subjects like magnetism and hydraulics as well as his specialist fields of styangraphy, palenchics and the caprimantic arts, whose scientific-sounding names concealed the fact that they were entirely of his own invention. He also put on demonstrations of electricity, frequently charging up and electrocuting the black cats he used in his displays.

His method of diagnosing influenza relied on his scientific know-how. Peering into the Solar Microscope, he claimed, he had been able to detect insects, 'seen as large as birds' nesting on hedges, which were responsible for the disease. According to Katterfelto the bugs swarmed over the city in a manner that bore comparison to the Italian plagues of 1423, a medical scare story by association if there ever was one. He claimed in 1783 that he himself had succumbed to the illness, but, by careful consultation of ancient texts, had managed to manufacture a cure that restored him to health in twelve hours. Katterfelto, the newspapers reported, 'as a philosopher and philanthropist', was willing to share this medicine with the public for a very reasonable five shillings a bottle. Orders flooded in, and even the King was intrigued.

For some reason though, the fortunes of Dr Katterfelto declined. Adverts appeared in the paper trying to sell off his scientific apparatus first for £2,500, reduced to a bargain £250 after a couple of months when no takers appeared. Allegations were made that his black cats were in fact devils, an accusation denied by Katterfelto in tones of sorrowful regret at the foolishness of the masses. As his credibility waned, he became a wandering mountebank, selling his nostrums and putting on scientific shows, not always to great success. He was imprisoned in Shrewsbury as a vagrant and at one of his demonstrations he managed to burn down a haystack when a fire balloon encountered navigation problems. Towards the end of his life he ended up in Whitby, where he delighted the locals by sticking his daughter to the ceiling with a giant magnet. He died in 1799 in Yorkshire.

Valentine Greatrakes was an Irish 'healer' born in 1628, known as the 'Irish stroker' because of his method of treatment. He would lay hands on his patients, curing them through his touch. He treated some famous patients in his day and an account of his life, including the 'strange cures' he performed, was published in 1666. This contains many testimonials to his powers, including one woman who, unable to get herself touched by him, drank instead some of his urine and poured it into her ears. Apparently this was enough to cure her of the stomach troubles she had been suffering with for years, as she voided four gallons of water and also much wind 'at her privy part'. Her previously distended belly shrank to three-quarters of a yard from its previous two, and her hearing was cured as well.

The Wisdom of Solomon

Dr Solomon was famous for his patent medicine Cordial Balm of Gold, which he proclaimed took nine weeks to make after laborious extraction of various choice balsams and some ultra-rare substance known as 'seed of gold'. It was actually nothing more mysterious than brandy, but garnered him a fortune and reputation sufficient to be amongst the first people cast for Madame Tussaud's original exhibition. Always on the lookout for a profit, on one occasion he charged each of his dinner guests two guineas at the end of the evening because they had all sampled some of his 'medicine'. He was eventually driven out of town after the husband of one of his patients discovered that his wife had taken such a liking to Dr Solomon's products that she was consuming bottles of the stuff. This was a situation he found repeated in the homes of his friends, so together they decided to revenge themselves on the doctor, setting upon

One quack (or quackess, in this case) was famous for her bone-setting capabilities. Sally or Sarah Mapp, also known as 'crazy Sally', was a bone-setter of prodigious strength. In her lifetime she became the acknowledged expert in the field, working in eighteenth-century London coffee houses. Her enormous girth signalled her extraordinary strength; she was able to reset a dislocated shoulder without any assistance and she effected seemingly miraculous cures, wrenching the backs of the bent straight and setting those with a limp on an even keel. She lived in some style, and swanked about in a gilded chariot with liveried servants, distributing handbills declaiming her prowess. Alas, she was also overfond of drink and frittered away her fortune, eventually dying in poverty in 1737 in Seven Dials.

him in a field and forcing him to drink his own wares. In chagrin at such treatment he went to live in Birmingham, returning later to his childhood home of Liverpool where he died in 1805.

The Chevalier Rides Out

John Taylor was the greatest oculist (eye specialist) of all, and even vies with sex quack James Graham for top seat in the quack hall of fame. Dubbing himself 'Chevalier', he was born in 1703 and during the course of his life gained entry into the highest ranks of European society. His autobiography, an epic of self-promotion and unlikely episodes, doesn't stand up as an accurate historical account of his life, but his career as quack and eye surgeon was widely recorded by contemporaries. He did have some skill in eye surgery, especially in treating cataracts, but his main gifts came in talking up his achievements and prowess. He claimed grand-sounding titles for himself – 'Opthalmiater Pontifical Imperial and Royal' was his favourite. Access to the crowned heads of Europe and even the Pope, whom he apparently lectured on theology and eyesight, was the fruit of his extraordinary skill as an oculist, he averred. He could in fact actually claim to be oculist to King George II, appointed in 1736, but his popularity wasn't as universal as he liked to boast. In Canterbury his coach was attacked by angry patients, and in Scotland rude tracts were published about him, castigating him for quackery and worse. One contemporary satire told of the 'Chevalier' cutting out pieces of his own buttocks and replacing the flesh with the eyes of his mother's pet dog. Taylor was such a quack he would, said the author, take out anyone's eyes and reinsert them back to front so any lady or gentleman could watch ideas passing in their own minds. It was worse still for the poor quack in Ireland, where the family of a boy he had blinded in a botched operation strung him upside down from the ceiling and tortured him, burning his head with flaming torches.

Taylor's showmanship was second to none. He would dress flamboyantly and travel with two coaches and six black

Not all his fellow doctors were impressed with Taylor, either. In France a Dr Lecat watched him operate on someone with a squint. Taylor, with typical bombast, tried to pass off a quackish explanation of his technique and promised to teach his fellow doctor his method. Dr Lecat saw through this smokescreen, however, and got even with the Chevalier. Inviting him to dinner, he served him with a human head split down the middle exposing the inner workings of the eyes, asking him again for an explanation of his technique. For once Taylor was struck dumb.

horses (five of which were reported to be blind due to their master's experiments). When addressing crowds he would speak in a strange garbled version of Latin, a concoction of his own which he called the 'true Ciceronean', throwing outrageous flattery and a hotchpotch of classical allusions into an incomprehensible mix. Something of a ladies' man, he claimed that he could see into the soul of any woman under forty, and had been inside more nunneries in Europe than any other man (always strictly for medical reasons). His surgical skills, he affirmed, could make the blind see again. He even wrote that he had cured the eighty-eight-year-old Johann Sebastian Bach of blindness, unconcerned that the great composer had died years before at the age of sixty-five.

Taylor wrote forty-five books, or so he said, in a variety of languages. His autobiography was the most famous, containing not only medical and ocular tales, but accounts of women Taylor had known, children he had fathered and, bizarrely, executions he had witnessed and assisted in around the world. Obviously under some instructions from his publisher to appeal to as wide an audience as possible, the mixture of sex and death made for an unconventional account of an eye surgeon's life. The book that perhaps best represents the bombastic nature of John 'Chevalier' Taylor is his volume – now sadly lost – *The Art of Making Love with Success*. He died in Prague in 1772, his business taken on by his son in London, who, though he shared his father's name, could not hope to match him in terms of showmanship.

'Dr' Saffold

Thomas Saffold was a famous quack of the seventeenth century, known for his tireless advertising. He described himself 'An Approved and Licensed Physician', and advertised his presence heavily through handbills along the Strand, Fleet Street and Whitehall. His advice was free, so long as patients bought some of his products, either pills or elixir. The medicines were little short of miracle products, or at least according to the advertising:

It's Saffold's Pills much better than the rest,
Deservedly have gain'd the name of Best:
In curing by the Cause, quite purging out
Of Scurvy, French Pox, Agues, Stone and Gout.

Alas, it seems he took his own claims too seriously, and when he fell ill in 1691 he refused all medical help other than his own pills. Needless to say, he soon passed away, a fact sarcastically noted by a local wit:

Here Lyes the corps of Thomas Saffold,
By Death, in spite of Physick, Baffl'd.

Saffold's business premises were taken over by John Case, another quack, who announced himself to the world with the catchy 'Within this place/Lives Doctor Case', a couplet *Tatler* reckoned made him more money than Dryden got from 'all his poetical works put together'.

Vote of Confidence

Joanna Stephens was a quack who achieved great fame in the first half of the eighteenth century. Her particular speciality was treating bladder and kidney stones, and the peak of her career came when she managed to con the whole

It was no surprise that men were keen to get hold of a new method for getting rid of bladder and kidney stones: traditional treatments consisted of 'cutting for the stone' or lithotomy. This involved puncturing the perineum with a knife deep enough to drain off the urine dammed up behind the offending stone. In pre-anaesthetic days this was an incredibly painful procedure, and men were usually only driven to it once the pain of their blocked urine built up to an unbearable level.

of the British nation into buying her secret remedies for 'the stone'.

A charming and astute saleswoman, Joanna courted powerful and influential people, including scientists and physicians who seemed completely duped by the wares she was peddling. At the height of her fame and reputation she announced that for a mere £5,000 she would disclose the secrets of her remedy to the British public, for the good of the nation's health. A subscription was immediately launched and money began to roll in from wealthy men, no doubt troubled by their own stone problems. Even the Prime Minister of the day made a contribution. Unfortunately, when it came to counting the money, only £1,365 had been raised. So great was the concern that Mrs Taylor's cures would be lost that Parliament appointed a commission to look into the matter. The commission (which contained some eminent medical men of the day) considered the business, declared themselves satisfied that the medicines were the real thing and recommended that the Government hand over the money, which they duly did. The details of the wonderful cures were revealed to an expectant public. There were three stock medicines. One contained eggshell and snails. Number two included herbs, honey and soap. Number three was a pill

In June 1876 a female quack was tried for conning a sovereign out of a pauper on the basis that she was the seventh daughter of a seventh daughter, and thus able to heal.

made of snails, carrots, burdock and other bits and pieces, all burnt until black. Bizarrely there was no public outcry at having paid for such useless concoctions. People carried on taking them for years, perhaps desperate to get some value for money. As for Joanna, she vanished, taking her £5,000 with her.

Let's Get This Show on the Road

Everyone knows what an American medicine man looks like, an image usually recalled from Westerns. Dressed in a top hat and frock coat, they address their audience from the back of their 'physick wagon', which serves as their home, transport and travelling dispensary. Assistants, who could be anything from Native Americans in full regalia, glamorous females or even a travelling musician or two, would help draw a crowd of curious townsfolk, and the 'doctor' would deliver the pitch for his snake-oil or miracle cure. This picture wasn't just a Hollywood confection; such characters really existed, and some were pretty successful.

Quacks in America could operate with relative freedom. As far back as 1511 Henry VIII had passed a law that tried to limit the activities of quacks in England, but for much of the nineteenth century con-men and rogue doctors could operate in America without too much fear of interference from the law. They certainly had a market ripe for exploitation. Towns were often many miles apart, and doctors were spread pretty thinly – anyone visiting town with a bottle of cure-all medicine was bound to do a good trade. After all, you could buy a stock and keep it in your cupboard against the day that illness struck – and you could also use it on your livestock, as many snake-oils claimed they could cure both man and beast. Nutrition was pretty poor in places as well, which gave any quack a good customer base of the frequently unwell; the pioneer diet, for example, relied heavily on salted pork, which had often fed on sewage and waste. Even teething babies were given bacon rind to chew on, often with a string attached so it could be retrieved if accidentally swallowed. Everybody drank alcohol, even small children, and hygiene wasn't at the top of anyone's agenda.

Preparing the Ground

Part of the attraction of the medicine show was that it appealed to people's enthusiasm for self-treatment. This was greatly encouraged by the Thomsonian medical movement, based on the teachings of a Mr Samuel Thomson, a hardcore herbalist. It held great sway in the US from the early 1800s. Key belief in his theory of medicine was that all illness was caused by the body lacking sufficient heat. Restore that, said Thomson, and illness would vanish. Treatments involved steam baths and the plant *Lobelia inflata*, charmingly known as 'puke weed'. Patients were wreathed in hot steam until they teetered on the brink of consciousness, and then fed the herbs, which would rapidly purge their system. Using this method Thomson and his growing army of herbal militants claimed that most diseases could be cured: cancer, VD, consumption and dysentery to name but a few.

Part of the appeal of Thomsonianism was the rejection of mainstream, regular doctors. The idea was that any man could become his own physician, and for $20 you could buy a complete system of his diagnoses and cures, as well as the right to practise as a Thomsonian physician. Convinced that they held the keys to healing, Thomsonians waged war on the medical establishment as elitist quacks, steeped in Latin and with the sole aim of harming their patients while relieving them of their cash. This anti-establishment rabble-rousing went down well, and tapped into an ethic of self-care already established in pioneers. Eventually the Thomsonians began to die out as regular medicine became more legislated.

Worming into the Market

'Dr' Thomas W. Dyott was one of the first great patent-medicine barons. Beginning as an apothecary's apprentice in England, he later moved to the US and opened a pharmacy in Philadelphia. His big-selling product was Robertson's Infallible Worm Destroying Lozenges, which earned him more that $250,000 in the 1820s. Inventing a medical past (he claimed he was the son of a fictitious Dr Robinson of Edinburgh), and conferring upon himself a degree to help sales along, he even built a model town for his employees. There they had to abide by a strict set of rules, including abstention from liquor, which sat oddly with the gallons of alcohol they were daily pouring into the patent medicines they manufactured. Bathing was also compulsory. Unfortunately a financial crisis in 1837 ended this utopian dream, and Dyott spent some time in prison.

Teepee Tonics

Native American medicine shows were a strange diversion on the quackery path. Settlers in America were fascinated by the indigenous people, and by the nineteenth century, the earlier antipathy was being replaced with an admiration for a people who were at one with nature. Indian remedy books were already available; titles included *The Indian Doctor's Dispensatory*, *The Indian's Guide to Health* and *The Indian Doctor's Practice of Medicine*. The stage was set, and it wasn't long before Indian patent medicines arrived on the market to cash in on this trend.

Most famous of all the Indian medicine brands was Kickapoo Indian Oil. The oil was, said the manufacturers, an ancient remedy handed down by wise medicine men, and contained an element so rare and strange that it defied all chemical analysis. Other Kickapoo products soon followed – Buffalo Salve, Kickapoo Indian Worm-Killer and the best-selling of all, Sagwa. Sold as a cure for both indigestion and rheumatism, it was in fact a powerful laxative, but would do white man heap good, and was beloved of Native Americans too. 'An Indian,' opined Buffalo Bill (brought in to lend some Wild West glamour to the product), 'would as soon be without his horse, gun, or blanket as without Sagwa.'

To promote and market their medicine, the two men behind the Kickapoo brand (so named because they thought it funny) opened a show in a tent outside the train station in Boston in 1881, moving to Cincinnati in 1887 and rechristening their tent the 'principal wigwam'. There they hired a warehouse, which people could visit to see 'real' Native Indian day-to-day life. Wigwams were pitched around the warehouse floor in a surreal attempt to recreate prairie life, and up to 800 Native Americans were hired to mill about in a manner designed to convince the public that this was a genuine snapshot of Indian life. When Native Americans weren't available, Irish labourers wearing make-up were recruited as stand-ins.

The Kickapoo shows were so successful that they eventually mutated into general vaudeville shows with an Indian flavour and strong product placement. Anything that got the crowds in was fine so long as they kept on selling the medicine. The business lasted until about 1912, when the owners sold it off to a new proprietor, but within two years it closed down. Other Indian medicine vendors had tried to get in on the act: Arizona Bill was a Welshman who didn't feel his valleys accent was an anomaly in one who claimed to have been raised by Indians after being snatched as an infant. (Apparently his audience wasn't bothered by this inconsistency either.) Another entrepreneur, Colonel T.A. Edwards, sold his Ka-Ton-Ka, an Indian cure-all alongside his other 'Indian' products Mox-i-tong and Quillaia soap, and developed a successful franchise operation.

Wizard Idea

John Hamlin was a travelling magician in the 1870s, and in his act he peddled a product called Wizard Oil, which he said would confer magician status on the purchaser. When a customer caught up with him one day, he feared the worst, assuming that the man had come to seek redress after the oil had failed to work. Instead the man told him that the Wizard Oil had actually cured his rheumatism. A light bulb appeared above Hamlin's head: he abandoned the magic act, and decided to go into the patent medicine business, roping in his brother to assist. Their first decision was to decide which ailments their product would cure; they made the sound choices of pneumonia, cancer and hydrophobia, as well as rheumatism. The formula for the oil apparently didn't require changing to gain these expanded powers – it still was 70 per cent alcohol, with camphor, cloves and turps amongst other ingredients.

Publicity was the key to ensuring good sales, and the Hamlins were diligent advertisers. They hired mobile troupes to go out around the American Midwest, setting up shows in town and selling the product from the wagon-cum-stage. The company also produced Wizard Oil songbooks, very cheap to buy and printed so that the audience could join in the songs at the medicine shows, the lyrics interspersed with lurid testimonials detailing the miraculous cures Wizard Oil had achieved.

Specialists

A popular medicine show con was the tapeworm scare. The showman would give a frightening account of a tapeworm, lodged inside the gut, followed by a list of symptoms they could cause and which were all deliberately general and vague: hunger, sleeplessness, tiredness and weakness. By now the listeners were beginning to suspect that they might have a worm; in fact, it was likely that many of them probably did due to poor sanitation and dirty meat. Some showmen had jars of pickled tapeworms displayed on stage, or hung up like bunting. Tapeworms were easy to procure from local slaughterhouses, and there was a company in Kansas that made artificial ones.

Once the audience was convinced that it had a great

worm chomping away in its guts, then the cures were introduced. Some were just laxative medicines, which might or might not dislodge a worm. One showman, 'Fabulous' Kelly, sold a version that was bright green and known as Shamrock Tapeworm Remover. Some quacks made pills with string inside; the pill was swallowed and dissolved in the stomach and eventually the piece of string emerged, wormlike. Others favoured the Murphy button, which had two halves that snapped together. If a piece of string had been concealed inside, the patient could be convinced that the button had somehow caught the worm when it emerged at the other end. If a patient was fortunate enough to actually pass a real worm then the quack would often bottle it and put it onstage with a label naming both its former host and the happy day of delivery.

Ray Black was a quack kidney specialist. He had travelled widely, and in Australia he was shown birds, so he said, that were 500 years old. To reach this great age they lived by springs where rare crystals formed, and Black was selling these same crystals, he claimed, to his audience. In reality they were just flavoured Epsom salts, but his technique was ingenious; his pitch dragged on so long that the audience began to get backache just standing there and listening to him. The power of suggestion was enough to convince them that this pain was kidney trouble, and they were snared into buying his wares.

Henry Gales sold a corn cure made of cellulose, which was no good for corns. From his platform he would carry out foot examinations, cutting off a person's corns and then displaying to the audience not the piece he had removed but a pieces of horse's hoof he had palmed earlier. No one could fail to be disgusted and amazed, and many were both. A ladies' man, he was eventually killed by the husband of a woman with whom he had eloped.

Cereal Killers

Two men, who though not strictly quacks, nonetheless harboured some very strange beliefs, which are now somewhat obscured behind the famous brands they launched. Sylvester Graham (1794–1851) was the inspiration behind the famous Graham Cracker and was opposed to many things – white bread, pork, tobacco, salt and condiments, all of which he thought detrimental to health. Most of all though, he hated sexual excess, especially masturbation. He preached that better health and control of sexual urges could be obtained through a proper diet. Meat especially was hazardous, as it inflamed the stomach, which in turn affected the other organs. Vegetarian diet and wholewheat foods were the best regime to ensure long life, a pronouncement that provoked an attack by a mob of angry butchers and bakers, convinced he was going to damage their livelihoods. John Harvey Kellogg (1852–1943) was actually a qualified doctor, and was admired for his surgical skill. However, he had some decidedly odd ideas about health and medicine. Like Sylvester Graham, he was ferociously anti-masturbation. He may have been anti-sex altogether: it is alleged that although married, he could never bring himself to consummate the union, believing it would be hazardous to his health. A vegetarian, he recommended a low-calorie diet and along with developing toasted flakes of wheat he is also credited with the creation of peanut butter. He was obsessed by the bowels, regarding them as the key to good health. Ninety per cent of illness, he claimed, came from poisons lurking in the colon. Patients at his sanatorium in Battle Creek were made to drink large amounts of water to flush their bowels, as well as having regular colonic irrigations. He himself was flushed out every day after breakfast. Bowls of yoghurt were prescribed, half to be eaten and the other half taken rectally. If that didn't cure the problem, Kellogg would remove a portion of offending bowel surgically, sometimes carrying out twenty procedures in one day. The toasted flakes of wheat Kellogg invented were later to become the famous cornflakes, although John Harvey was only interested in them for their place in the diet of his patients. It was his more entrepreneurial brother William Keith Kellogg who took the flakes, tinkered with the recipe, and sold them to the world.

POTIONS, PILLS AND MACHINES

How far will people go for a cure? Judging by some of the bizarre remedies and contraptions that have been used over the centuries, pretty far. The great quack machine age from about 1850 to 1950 saw devices so ridiculous the mind boggles that anyone could have believed they would ever work, let alone cure them. That it took appearances in law courts to get some of them removed from sale is even more surprising. Consider, for example, one Victorian device: Bellhouse's patent Anti-Rheumatic Towel. Simply drying off after a bath with this magical cloth would prevent, according to the adverts, 'rheumatism, neuralgia, constipation, indigestion, and liver complaints'. Bizarre pills, potions and lotions have all figured in the irregular medicine chest, and sometimes worse, as in the case of the two Mozambicans who were recently arrested in possession of a pair of human testicles. They were charged with the murder of the owner, from whom they had removed the gonads to sell to a witch doctor to use as *muti*, a traditional medicine.

QUACK MAGIC

 Although *muti* is a South African word that means traditional medicine, more recently it has become associated with pagan or occult rituals. It is based on the idea of taking the energy of another living thing as your own. Most of the time the power of plants, herbs or animals is enough, but sometimes only a human will do. Children are thought to have the most power, as they have not yet been contaminated by adult life. Different body parts are used in medicines, depending on what is required; a heart, for example, might be used to increase courage, while eyeballs might be used to improve failing sight. Chillingly, body parts are thought most powerful if they are removed while their victim is still alive.

Fatal Attraction

Magnets have been used in medicine for hundreds of years, their rise to popularity beginning almost as soon as someone pulled the first lodestone (rocks containing magnetite) from the ground. With their ability to mysteriously attract iron, these magnetic stones were almost inevitably ascribed magical powers. Unsurprisingly, by the Middle Ages, physicians had claimed them as medical miracles: lodestones were touted as an aphrodisiac, and had the happy side effect of curing ailments like gout, arthritis, poisoning and baldness as well. People seemed happy enough to believe in the magic pebbles for a while and Paracelsus made it his work to investigate whether magnetic rocks could treat epilepsy, diarrhoea, haemorrhages and other assorted complaints.

One of the most famous quacks of all was a man who made his fortune through magnetism – Franz Anton Mesmer. Born in 1734 he was sincere but misguided, a zealous believer in his own theories. He developed his pet philosophy of animal magnetism from his belief that the stars could affect changes in man through their influence on an invisible 'fluidum' that ran through the universe and every living body. A respectable doctor when he developed this theory, he was attracted to the work of the sinister-sounding Dr Hell, who was at that time using magnets in his treatment of patients. Mesmer, bolting his theories on to the work of this doctor, became convinced that magnets would have an effect on the fluid that coursed through everyone. He would be able to cure patients with magnets too! After trying his theories on patients in Vienna he became convinced that he did not need magnets to cure people – rather, the power lay within himself. He would be able to magnetise anything, from a loaf of bread to his pet dog. This was all too much for the local Viennese medical establishment who didn't want to be seen harbouring eccentric quacks and he was ordered to leave town. He went to set up in Paris, arriving in 1778. His methods brought immediate acclaim. He opened a luxurious salon where patients would come to stand around impressive 'magnetic tubs', fitted with iron conductors and rods. First they would press their knees against those of their neighbour to convey the animal magnetism. Next the assistant magne-tisers appeared, young men who would massage the breasts and thighs of the (mainly female) patients gently until they reached some sort of hysterical crisis. Mesmer would then enter the room. He would wear a lilac suit, wave a white wand and play a harmonica to set the mood, then wander the room touching his patients with his wand and staring piercingly into their eyes. Once the 'crisis' had passed, the patients were released. However, once again Mesmer was run out of town after a commission investigated his activities and pronounced that 'animal magnetism' was a load of quackish rubbish, and his cures had instead been affected by some unknown physiological cause. If he had started with genuine medical beliefs, it appears that Mesmer had lapsed into quackery, and he died in 1815 having all but abandoned medicine in favour of playing his glass harmonica.

For a while magnetism as a medical cure lost its attraction,

One of the first household quack devices ever invented relied on magnetism. Dr Perkins operated in the USA in the eighteenth century. In 1796 he applied for a patent for his 'metallic tractors'. These were metal rods made of brass and iron, about three inches long. The idea was that the patient was to draw out disease by rubbing their affected parts with the tractors. The whole thing was based on Luis Galvani's theory of animal electricity, which Perkins had eagerly absorbed. (Galvani had demonstrated how an electrical current made a frog's leg twitch in 1786.) Receiving little support from his professional brethren, Perkins nonetheless entered into the manufacture of his tractors, and soon found himself riding the wave of a craze. Even George Washington himself bought a pair. Despite being thrown out of the Connecticut Medical Society to which he belonged for being a 'user of nostrums', Perkins carried on selling like there was no tomorrow (£10 per pair, half price for medical professionals and free to the clergy) and even opened a branch office in England, where business was initially brisk. However, all good things must end, and sales of the tractors fell away, leaving Perkins with a need for a new product. He duly concocted a remedy for the dreaded yellow fever. It was certainly cheap to make, containing only vinegar and muriate of soda, and was about as useful as the ingredients suggest. Perkins took some off to New York during a fever outbreak to prove its worth. Unfortunately it was useless and Perkins himself caught the fever and died in 1799.

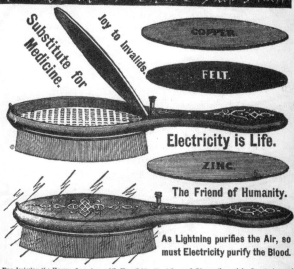

but the nineteenth and twentieth centuries saw a rash of quack magnetic devices and cures come on the market. Magnetic insoles for the shoes would guarantee warm feet and ward off illness – by increasing the circulation in the feet the magnetic pieces would stop headaches caused 'by too much blood on the brain'. Magnetic hatbands had the advantage of both increasing memory power and preventing baldness. And all for $2.50 in 1908. Magnetic belts and corsets would help the bearing and digestion, and lung protectors would strengthen these vital organs against invading airborne illness. The public eagerly snapped up anything that was imbued with this mysterious force, and quacks had a field day.

Lightning Cures

Electricity was the other natural force that proved a boon to quack doctors. Not only would it provide power to drive some of the ludicrous machines they were selling as medical devices, but it was also a valuable commodity on the medicine market in itself. One quack got in on the act early. 'Count' Mattei sold electrical remedies at the end of the nineteenth century. Advertised everywhere, the 'Count' had three specific remedies patriotically created in the colours of the Italian flag – Electricita Bianca, Rossa and Verde. Upon investigation, however, these phials of liquid held no magnetic or electrical powers; just plain water.

But the Count's failure didn't matter, for the electrical age of quackery was in full swing. Electricity appealed to quacks because to the layman it appeared magical – invisible forces able to turn motors, and power machines. Quacks could pretend they had harnessed this invisible sorcery for medical benefit, and sell it on as a cure. One advantage that electricity did have was that you could actually feel it; give someone a small jolt and they will feel an instant effect, something taking a medicine could rarely achieve.

Electrical medical machines therefore became very popular for a time. These included devices like electric corsets, sold to women to provide invigoration to their whole system when they wore them. 'A Boon to Women', said the adverts, promising that any woman who wore one would be free from hysteria, dyspepsia and all 'rheumatic and organic infections'. The corsets were advertised by pen illustrations of ladies in various states of undress, no doubt to capture the browsing eye of any husbands who happened to be leafing through their wife's periodicals.

Electric belts were also popular, aimed at men who might be suffering from all manner of afflictions. Weak kidneys, bladder trouble, the worryingly vague 'early decay' and a host of other complaints could be effectively dispelled through wearing an electrical belt. The pictures showed robust young men, stripped to their long johns and wearing the belts, out of which showered sparks in all directions. 'I am a man once more,' thundered the muscle-bound gent who featured on the adverts for the Supreme Electric Belt. These belts, many with clip-on additions and 'suspensory sacks' in which men could swaddle their testicles for a jolt of electrical treatment, flooded the market.

However, quacks didn't stop there. Where Elisha Perkins had initially blazed the trail with his electric tractors, others were keen to follow. Between about 1860 and 1920, electrical medical paraphernalia enjoyed its heyday, and all manner of weird and wonderful devices hit the market, to be snapped up by a public blinded by a little science and a lot of false

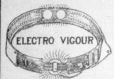

promises. Electrical rings, designed to draw out illness by extracting the disease in the blood, were popular, and tapped into a tradition of medical finger pieces going back centuries.

For women (and men) who gained a taste for electrical jewellery, a medallion or pendant was also available, which, worn around the neck, would confer electrically charged good health. Batteries could be purchased, which could be strapped directly on to the skin allowing electricity to course all over the body (in the adverts, at least) spreading health and well-being wherever it went. Personal adornment with fashionable electrical jewellery was complemented by electrical grooming products. A popular sideline with manufacturers of bogus medical devices was the electric brush. Often this was a battery to which a variety of devices could be attached – combs, brushes, rollers and sponges. The home consumer could then apply these to themselves wherever necessary in the privacy of their own home, for an impressive list of complaints. Offering hope for the bald in 1872, Dr Scott's Electric Brush promised to cure headaches both bilious and nervous, as well as preventing baldness, dandruff and greyness, and all for a few shillings. Only to be used by the purchaser, each box warned 'in no case should more than one person use the brush. If always used by the same person it retains its full curative power.' One brush per household wouldn't do anything for profits.

Perhaps the most overreaching piece of electrical quackery was the 1932 Rejuvenator. Like an iron lung, patients would lie down inside while combinations of infra-red and ultra-violet lights shone upon the patient. Not used for any specific disease, the Rejuvenator had much grander claims – it could prolong youth and even reverse the ageing process. For such a huge scientific breakthrough the results were somewhat

QUACK MAGIC

The Electropoise was electrical quackery at its finest, first hitting the market in 1893. Consisting of a cylinder, the Polizer, attached by a wire to a metal disc, the instrument was designed to introduce electricity to the body. The disc, attached to the skin, would be charged by the Polizer, allowing oxygen to be absorbed through the pores. Impressive-sounding stuff, only slightly spoiled by the fact that the Polizer was just a hollow piece of painted gas pipe. That the human body cannot absorb oxygen through the skin is merely incidental. Enough people bought an Electropoise to give its inventor, Hercules Sanche, the encouragement to devise another money-spinner, the Oxydoner. This was essentially the same device as the Electropoise, except this time the Polizer was dunked in a bowl of water to do its work. A model for couples was developed, so they could both wire themselves up before retiring for the night, and an owners' club was also convened, which allowed purchasers of the machines to meet and swap stories of their miracle cures. So enthusiastic were these consumers that Sanche somehow managed to persuade them to give him money, 'convertible donations', which he could use at his own discretion. Last heard of in the 1940s, Dr Sanche went to his grave an unrepentant quack.

A more recent piece of quackery involved motorcycle daredevil Evel Knievel, who appeared on American TV advertising a painless electrical cure called the Stimulator. Evel testified (for a reputed $10,000 per week) that simply by holding the device against any part of his body the pain there would melt away. How this was happening is a mystery, since the Stimulator was no more than an electric gas oven lighter, battery powered and emitting a low voltage spark. The Food and Drug administration soon stepped in and in 1997 the company was forced to refund customers who had bought Stimulators as hugely inflated prices.

disappointing. The inventor of the machine, W.E. Mortrude, was declared bankrupt shortly after launching his enterprise and his machines disappeared from public view.

Doctor on the Radio

Radionics is a branch of medicine exclusively the preserve of quacks. The founding father of this esoteric discipline is one Dr Albert Abrams, who qualified as a regular doctor in 1882. However, it seems he soon wearied of this work, and decided to explore the exciting world of fringe medicine. Unsure of what discipline to follow, Dr Abrams hit on the idea of inventing his own speciality, which he called spondylo-therapy. Now he had created this new field of medicine he decided it needed a canon, so Abrams wrote a book about it, which proved a great success and went through many editions. Encouraged by the reaction to his creation, he started giving lessons in spondylotherapy at $200 per course. What the eager disciples on these courses learned was vague. Spondylotherapy was based on percussion of the spine, which seemed to involve tapping away at the back. Even Dr Abrams didn't appear entirely at home with his new medical system, because he soon abandoned the spine in favour of the abdomen. Key to this change in location was the new medical diagnostic machine that the ever-inventive Abrams had developed – the Dynamizer. This amazing new medical tool was indeed a remarkable machine. A drop of blood was taken from a patient and put on a piece of blotting paper inside the machine. A wire went from the machine to the forehead of a healthy person, who stood facing west in a dim light, stripped to the waist. Dr Abrams then tapped away at this person's abdomen, mapping out areas of 'dullness' on this diagnostic sounding board, until he eventually produced an analysis of the blood sample in the Dynamizer. This technique caught on, helped by the wide-eyed innocence with which people viewed technology. Dr Abrams soon claimed that he could even tell a person's religion by the sample they provided, which didn't need to be a blood sample – a simple signature would suffice. Dressing the whole thing up in pseudoscientific mumbo-jumbo, Abrams talked loftily about SV reactions and VR6 conductive energy.

However, Abrams wasn't content with just diagnosing people's illnesses, not when there was money to be made in providing them with cures as well. Thus the Ossilloclast was born. This machine, claimed the doctor, cured through vibratory impulses, just as drugs did. In a radical new interpretation of how pharmaceuticals actually worked, untroubled by scientific evidence, Abrams stated that drugs worked because they had the same vibrating frequency as the disease they cured. Therefore his amazing new Ossilloclast, which could be set to vibrate at many different speeds, could cure all diseases through the transmission of invisible radio waves. The machine was a licence to print money. Not available for sale, Abrams leased them out to practitioners for $250 per year plus a $200 correspondence training course. Anyone who signed up had to swear they would never open a machine to see how it worked. When he died in 1923 Abrams had stashed away over $2m.

When tested by a scientific panel, Abrams's machine failed to work.. He blamed this breakdown on the sceptical nature of the investigators, whose negative thoughts, he claimed, were affecting his delicate electronic equipment.

POTIONS, PILLS AND MACHINES

Of course, the jealous men who made up the mainstream medical profession failed to appreciate the medical advances that Abrams was making, and were intent on discrediting his vibratory gospel. One doctors sent in some guinea-pig's blood to be diagnosed by Dynamizer. The results came back that the patient had 'general cancer and tuberculosis of the genito-urinary tract'. Another sent in some sheep's blood, which came back with the unfortunate tidings that it was suffering from hereditary syphilis. The American Medical Association managed to obtain a machine, and against all the rules opened it up; inside were electrical components randomly connected to one another.

Although Abrams was dead, radionics didn't die with him. Instead it was taken up by other quacks, who seized on the idea of medical radio waves as a way of tuning into the frequency of a quick buck. First amongst these was Ruth Drown, dubbed the 'queen of quacks'. Dr Ruth Drown claimed she could diagnose and treat disease with her patent devices, Drown Radio Therapy and Drown Radio Vision Instruments (also known as 'Homo-Vibra Ray Instruments).

These devices were similar to those of Abrams. They tuned in to the 'vibrations' of the body, and could locate and identify not only disease, but gauge blood pressure, examine urine and sample the temperature of the patient. When her devices and technique were put to independent test, however, she failed spectacularly. She was unable to diagnose any illnesses accurately from provided blood samples of patients, instead preferring to find as much trouble in as many parts of the body as possible, hoping to register at least one lucky guess. Undeterred, Mrs Drown opened an institute in Los Angeles – the Drown College – where she taught her methods. She also made a fair profit from selling her quack machines. There were home kits for people to use for self-treatment, bigger pieces of apparatus for use in surgeries and even a long-distance machine, which could be used to treat patients remotely. All the practitioner needed was a sample of blood on which to work. Unfortunately, most of these devices were either empty of all circuitry, or filled with junk electronic components that were badly connected. When Mrs Drown died in 1962 she was waiting to go to court for her second fraud trial.

George de la Warr picked up the radionics baton in England. Born in 1904, he took to building radionic 'Black Boxes'. Amongst his numerous medical claims for his devices he also added agricultural applications. Simply by smearing a photo of a farm with insecticide and putting it into one of his machines, he said, he could kill pests in a field miles away.

Ore-Inspiring Radiation Cures

Radiation wasn't always the feared substance it is nowadays. Forget nuclear bombs, fallout and Chernobyl; radiation was once sold as a healthy product and a cure for diseases. Around the turn of the century, people began to get interested in radiation even if they didn't really understand it. What they did know about it all sounded good; it emanated energy, glowed in the dark, and could help treat illnesses like

Radium was believed to cure all sorts of diseases, including constipation, hay fever, typhoid, eczema, arthritis and hundreds of others.

A chocolate bar, laced with radium, was sold in the 1920s. Like Mortrude's 1930s machine, it was called the Rejuvenator.

cancer. It was this last benefit that really captured the imagination of the public, and soon all sorts of radiation-containing products were flooding the market.

Bogus quack products, trading on the health-giving benefits of radium, quickly flooded the market. One of the most popular items was the radioactive water jar. With names such as Health Fountain and Vitalizer, this product promised health-imbibing radioactive water in every home. The jar was lined with radioactive ore to infuse the water, which was topped up every day, usually to far above today's recommended radioactive limits. The most popular model was the Revigator, which sold hundreds of thousands of models until the 1930s, when concerns about radiation led to a rapid drop in sales.

Other quacks saw a connection between radiation and health and developed a whole range of ore-containing products aimed at the public. Radioactive ointments like the 1920 Linarium promised to bring the user relief from sore muscles and joints. 'Throw away canes and bandages. Feel young and active again,' claimed the adverts. Sex cures also proliferated. Some, like Arium, hinted at renewed vitality and vigour for men and women. Others, like the scary sounding Glands and Radium, were far more direct. These pills were a potent mixture, according to the manufacturers, of the still-warm glands of animals, mixed with radium salts. Glands and Radium could be taken as tablets and used in conjunction, for even better results, with radioactive suppositories! Once the nuclear rod had been inserted into the rectum (or vaginally) the radiation would be absorbed by the surrounding tissue over the next few days with the happy results of not only boosting flagging sex drive, but also clearing up any local problems like piles, incontinence and inflammation. What was done with the spent nuclear waste is unclear.

Ray Therapy

Healing rays are the half-brother of medicinal radiation, and have been accompanied by as much confusion and quackery as their sibling. One of the first great 'ray therapies' was the blue-glass cure, first promoted by an old civil war general, A.J. Pleasonton, in 1861. The General believed that light which had passed through blue glass could somehow halt illness and restore health in both man and beast, an idea expounded in his treatise written, of course, with blue ink on blue-tinted paper 'in an attempt to relieve the eyes of the

A medical historian has revealed that blue-glass therapy came about as a result of a botched order in a glass-making firm. Having produced far too much blue glass, the firm asked a salesman if he could get rid of the surplus. After a conversation with a scientific friend, who jokingly remarked that blue might cure disease, the salesman hit upon the idea of selling all his glass as a cure for aches and pains. He sent some to General Pleasonton, who allowed the sun to shine through the glass on to his old war wounds. Remarkably, he found himself much fortified by this treatment. The General was a well-known public figure, and with thousands of wounded Civil War veterans looking for a treatment for old wounds, the newspapers covered the story of this remarkable discovery and the orders soon flooded in.

reader'. Popular songs were, penned about the General's wonder cure, but the fad for blue glass passed away.

Electricity, and particularly electric light, gave a boost to ray therapy. In the 1930s the Spectro-Chrome was effectively a lamp with some coloured slides. Patients could either be treated at home or at the 'doctor's'. They would sit naked in front of the machine and be bathed in coloured lights for various conditions. It was also important that the patient observed the correct lunar cycles before undergoing treatment, as the correct phase of the moon was crucial for a successful cure. Spectro-Chrome therapy was the brainchild of 'Dr' Dinash Ghadiali. Although he didn't have any medical qualifications he did have an impressive criminal record with convictions for fraud, kidnap, 'illicit relations' and running illegal operations. Nonetheless, by 1940 his quackery had brought him over $1m. He died in 1966, but his son today carries on his work.

Other ray devices also flourished. Ultra-violet rays were extremely popular with quacks and all sorts of different useless devices were manufactured for myriad complaints. Generally they were devices containing an electrical coil that could produce a blue (violet) spark, which was completely harmless. Violet ray rakes were sold for running through the thinning locks of the bald in the hope they would stimulate some tonsorial activity. Wart and spot removers were extremely popular, and one manufacturer claimed his product could eliminate freckles and treat obesity. Some were designed with prongs, which fitted up each nostril, to remove unsightly hair, while others were to be inserted into any orifice available. Ear devices, for example, used violet rays 'for treating deafness . . . ringing in the ears and earache'. The instructions for rectal and vaginal probes were less detailed.

Help-to-Hear

Quack cures for the deaf and blind litter the landscape, like the eyes of Dr T.J. Eckleburg. Devices like the 1903 Help-to-Hear could be found in the back of any magazine, and could be bought via mail order for just a few dollars. In the case of this device, the inventor claimed to have discovered a simple device, which would allow even the most profoundly deaf person to hear. He himself, who had been deaf for twelve years, could bear witness to the extraordinary properties of the device. Who couldn't be swayed by such a convincing argument? People sent off their money and received back through the post a small sheet of hard rubber. This they were supposed to hold against their front teeth, pointing towards the sound. It hardly warranted scientific investigation to decide that the Help-to-Hear was completely useless. The hapless manager of the company was prosecuted, admitting in court that he had never in fact been deaf and that the pieces of rubber he sold for $2 cost him 7 cents each. The company was declared fraudulent and closed in 1906.

Patent ear oils were also popular deafness cures, designed to be poured into the ear canal to relieve deafness. Catarrh was widely held to be a cause of hearing loss, and quacks concentrated on this area. Products like Stuart's Catarrh tablets – 'We KNOW that regular daily use of these

Claxton's patent Ear-Cap had a number of bonuses: 'remedying prominent ears, preventing disfigurement in afterlife, keeps the hair tidy'. Prospective purchasers in 1872 were to send their head measurement and 3s 6d to an address in the Strand.

tablets will cure catarrh' – and devices like the Blowena concentrated on relieving deafness through the elimination of the insidious build-up of matter. In the case of the latter, the patient would put one end in their mouth, the other up their nose, and literally blow away their hearing problems!

Quacks had a field day with eyesight too. Ointments, eye machines and dubious therapeutic drills were all aggressively marketed. The first patent was registered in 1851 by Jonathan Ball for his ivory eye massagers. Some quacks even introduced eye tests, which deliberately gave the impression that there was a problem with someone's eyesight when in fact there was none. Blindness cures have a long history. During Restoration times, England was a hotbed of quackery, drawing in all sorts of rogue doctors from Europe. One of the most famous of these was Cornelius Tilburg. He based his medical practice on the 'no cure, no fee' principle, and he claimed medical success in an impressive array of fields: kidney stones, recovering sight to the blind, deafness, vomiting, 'rising of the vapours' and all 'scorbutick distempers' were just some of his specialities. He illustrated his expertise by publishing lists of people he had successfully cured, and of what disease: 'Mr Christopher Shelly was brought to me in a chair, deprived of all his limbs, incapable of moving hand or foot was (by the blessing of God) perfectly cured by me.' Setting himself up near Covent Garden, he specialised in restoring the sight of the 'stone-blind', while still offering cures for rupture and those who had been at 'Venus sports' and contracted any variety of venereal disease. As a sideline he took up cosmetic dentistry with the enchanting invitation to those with dirty teeth – 'although they be black as pitch [I can] make them extraordinary white'. He was succeeded in his practice by his son James, described as a 'famous outlandish Doctor', who also specialised in treating those who may have 'anchored in a strange harbour' and caught the French pox.

'Professor' Samuels came along a few hundred years later with his patent eye water. Not only claiming to cure blindness, he claimed he could, via the eyeballs, cure consumption, fits, heart trouble and many more diseases simply through the application of his wondrous eye water. Branded an 'unconscionable scoundrel' by the medical profession, his eye water was nothing more than a salt and sugar solution.

Eye exercisers were a quackish mainstay. These could be devices that patients could use on themselves, or a regimen of exercises, which, if followed, were supposed to restore the sight. Products like the American Dr J. Stephens Patent Cornea Restorer from 1865 promised to 'render spectacles useless', and were joined on the shelves by such useless machines as the Neu-Vita Oculizer, which operated by poking the eyes with rubber prods, and the Natural Eye Normalizer, which worked by slightly twisting the eyelids. This last product was finally removed from the shelves in 1937 by a fraud trial. One of the most famous ideas to enjoy popularity for a while was 'palming', literally pressing the eye with the hand to somehow restore the sight. Devoted to this was Aldous Huxley, whose eyesight was so bad he was only able dimly to perceive this world, let alone the brave new one round the corner. He fell for the quackish pronouncements of W.H. Bates, whose 1920 opus *Better Sight Without Glasses* is still on sale today. Bates recommended 'palming' as a way of obtaining better vision, and although pushing the eyeball does temporarily change the shape of the lens and so affect eyesight, it has no permanent effect.

POTIONS, PILLS AND MACHINES

Exercise for Better Health

Some machines, which were sold under the delusion that they would bring some medical benefit, seem, these days, utterly ridiculous. One of these was the Vigor's 1867 Horse Action Saddler. Highly approved by no less personages that His Imperial Majesty the Emperor of Austria and His Royal Highness the Prince of Wales, these bizarre (and quite large) devices were recommended for a range of medical complaints, including: poor circulation; ill-functioning liver; hysteria; insomnia; gout; dyspepsia; and rheumatism. The Horse Action Saddler was in fact a mechanical indoor horse, which could be set to trot, canter or gallop, depending on the level of exercise required. Advertisements showed a frock-coated gentleman with ramrod-straight back accompanied by a lady, decorously riding side-saddle in a model of Victorian propriety, enjoying a swift canter in their drawing room. If any were not swayed by this impressive scene, respected medical journal The *Lancet* added its voice: 'the expense and difficulty of riding a live horse are avoided'.

Reast's Invigorator Belt was one of the few belts on the market at the time that wasn't electrical. It was recommended for those with postural problems to provide, 'an upright,

One nineteenth-century advert featured a man, for some reason wearing a bow tie, lying in bed with a hose protruding out from under the covers. Under the bed was mass of machinery, which, when activated, pumped steam up the pipe and under the bedclothes. 'A thorough Turkish Hot Air and vapour bath for 3d,' was the explanation for this strange scene.

soldierly bearing', beloved of ladies and sons of empire. Many of the electrical belts manufactured actually had no electrical current whatsoever – instead the insides were smeared with a mixture of glue and pepper, so the wearer would feel a 'tingle' when they put it on.

Carter's literary machine (patent, of course) was one of a range of items of invalid furniture. Essentially it was a book holder, which enabled those bound to the bed or bath-chair to study the page without the added burden of actually having to hold the book. All for £1 1s. Also available, for indigestion, were exercise chairs with horse action at a more expensive £5 5s.

Bad Medicine

Patent medicine, snake-oil, wonder cures and miracle drugs are the quack's stock-in-trade. Quacks and doctors have always relied on their potions and medicines as a vital way of relieving their patients of illness and money, not necessarily in that order. Their manufacture could range from gathering

Worm exterminator Pulvis Benedictus was a powerful quack medicine, which required a book of fifteen chapters to describe its wonderful powers. Testimonials played an important part, like that of Mr Stiles of Smithfield who was practically consumed alive by an eight-foot worm, a fate he could have avoided if only he had taken the exterminator. Mr Stubbs was reported of having an unusual experience when 'about to embalm a Gentlewoman who had been dead eight and forty hours. When working his operation, her heart leapt out upon the table, and out of it he took a worm as thick as an arrow, with two heads, one like a serpent.'

herbs growing in fields to knocking up dubious alchemical mixtures containing any number of esoteric ingredients. Some were effective, later to provide the basis for 'proper' medicines, like the use of foxgloves to cure dropsy. Others were more exotic; concoctions mixing sulphur, gold and arsenic were considered by some scholars to be able to confer longevity on whoever drank them.

The term 'patent medicine' came from mid-eighteenth-century England where the King granted, for a fee, royal patents for products. The patents protected the ownership rights of the products and also conferred some prestige to the medicines, but some medicines became famous in their own right: Bile Beans, Morrison's Vegetable Pills, Dover's Powders and Pink Pills for Pale People all sold well without the benefit of a royal patent. A patent wasn't any guarantee that a medicine would work: all that was required to gain one was proof that it was an original formula.

Patent medicines weren't strictly the preserve of out-and-out quacks though. 'Proper' doctors saw the profits that their irregular brethren were turning and decided to get in on the act as well. Nehemiah Grew, for example, was a regular eighteenth-century doctor, who patented his own medicine, Epsom Salts. Dr Hans Sloane promoted medicinal chocolate. From the mid-seventeenth century, there were literally hundreds of patent products to choose from, for all kinds of complaints. Pills like Peter's Famous Head Pill promised to cure convulsions and 'Apoplectick fits'. If a person was to

Robert Turlington was one of the first people to receive a patent in the 1740s for his medicine, Balsam of Life.

take it even just once every twenty days it would ensure that they remained in good health, 'for it resists all putrefaction, and will continue good some Seven years or more'. Children with worms were advised to take Jones's Friendly Pill, which apparently worked in 'seven several ways' to rid them of the unwanted guests and also purged 'so gentle'. Dr Case sold a Cordial Elixir, which overcame scurvy by 'opening obstructions to the spleen, and purging melancholy humours from the blood'. Scot's Pills were available as a general tonic, especially good after hard drinking, according to the label. Anodyne necklaces were something of a quackish mainstay. Sold by a Dr Choke in the seventeenth century, they were also touted by a Dr Tanner, Dr Burchell and Dr Chamberlen. These 'Miraculous' necklaces were beads of peony wood on a string, and were recommended for teething children, who were to be dressed in them from two months old until all their teeth were cut. Apart from making teething painless and easy the necklaces were also said to guard against epilepsy, a Roman idea.

Some products traded on healthy-sounding, although rather vague, claims, such as Vogeler's Curative Compound. Billed as a 'blood purifier and strength restorer' for all diseases of the blood and stomach, it could also cure melancholia, hysteria, eczema, headaches and 'debility'. The efficacy of this wonderful potion was attested to by a Mrs

Powdered mummy was used for a variety of illnesses ranging from asthma to poisoning. Eventually its use declined in the seventeenth century when the pain and vomiting it induced became too much for people to bear.

POTIONS, PILLS AND MACHINES

One seventeenth-century cure was well named – the Perpetual Pill. Made of antimony, it was a powerful laxative, which would pass through the system quickly. When it emerged at the other end it could be washed off and used again.

Lilian Smith of 21 Cambridge Road, Walthamstow, whose case history appeared in the advertising: 'for nine years afflicted with nervous prostration, hysteria, dyspepsia and congested kidneys: was completely cured after taking four bottles of Vogeler's Curative Compound'.

Cosmetic Medicine

Quackish potions excelled in the beauty market. The pursuit of beauty has proved a lucrative area for quacks to exploit. While quacks got men to buy their various devices and potions by playing on their fears of impotence and lack of manly 'vigour', women were targeted over concern about their appearance. Particularly profitable were obesity cures, a market that today is even bigger business. At the turn of the century, quacks would think nothing of advertising miracle products designed to make the bloated svelte again. You could, for example, buy a tin of patent Fatoff Obesity Cream. All you had to do was rub some into the flabby skin every night and just watch the fat melt away. Kellogg's sold a box of Safe Fat Reducer, claiming that it could 'reduce you to a normal weight safely, without starvation diet or tiresome exercises'. In fact it was anything but safe, being comprised of toast and thyroid extract, which should only be taken under the supervision of a real doctor. Sticking to cornflakes was probably safer. Allan's Anti-Fat was another product available to portly Victorians, which claimed

Quacks often produced handbills, which promised much of their potions and remedies. In 1677 The Woman's Prophecy offered relief from 'The Glimmering of the Gizard, the Quavering of the Kidneys and the Wambling Trot'.

to stop the stomach changing food into fat. If you weren't convinced then turning to Trilene – 'the only stoutness cure' – might work. After all, as a Mrs Fenton from Tydsely testified, 'Been fat all my life, but now your tablets tell a tale. I have lost 17lb already, and am delighted.'

The eighteenth century had already seen an explosion in beauty medicines, especially because of the prevalence of smallpox, which ruined and pitted complexions. Remedies like Balsamick Essence were targeted at women whose countenance was showing signs of wear and tear: after all, if women were not pleasing to look upon, warned the advertisements, then their husbands would be 'offended at their deformities and turn to others'. Special washes were available from gentlewoman quacks, which promised to flush away all redness, pimples, yellowness and freckles. Grey or red hair (which was considered undesirable) could be changed to 'a lovely brown, which never decays, changes, or smoots the linnen'. Lurking in a London coffee house, the inventor of World's Beautifyer could be consulted on the removal of red faces in men or women, whereas the Water of Talk and Pearl was sold by several rivals to those who wanted to achieve anything from removing their wrinkles to growing back the hair on a bald head.

Ladies again were the target when it came to hair – either too much or not enough. 'Ladies, don't shave,' implored the manufacturers of the Floral Depilatory. Similarly the Capillus

Most quack hair growth and restorative products contained lead or arsenic, which indeed would make the hair look darker and thicker for a while. Unfortunately, it could also poison.

company promised to rid women of superfluous hair, with a treatment that rather ominously promised no hair would ever sprout again where its product had touched. Women who had the opposite problem of not having enough were advised to turn to products like Tressalena, which depicted on its label a woman who on one side of her scalp had the cropped hairstyle of a convict ready for deportation and on the other the long flowing locks of the Victorian ideal. Men, who were worried by the 'alarming increase in baldness', noted by the Edwards Harlene Co. of Holborn, were relieved to find that they produced a remedy for this condition, 'a Great Hair producer and Restorer'.

Even foodstuffs had medical claims attached to them. Cadbury's Cocoa was sold on the basis of its bodybuilding properties; it was billed 'the strongest in Flesh formers'. Adverts depicted a doctor in his surgery prescribing it to a nubile young woman. Tomato ketchup even started its life as a patent medicine – Dr Miles's Compound Extract of Tomato. This was something of a comeback for the tomato, which had at one time been regarded as a deadly poison. Even coffee had its day as a medicine, widely prescribed for a variety of complaints in the eighteenth century.

Patent medicines didn't die out abruptly at the end of the nineteenth century, as the demonic sounding 666 Tonic demonstrates. Adverts from 1918 show that the market for this remedy for headaches, biliousness, loss of appetite, foul breath and aching was still there. The price was one soul.

QUACK MAGIC

In 1906, legislation in the USA put paid to many patent medicines as it required that they reveal their ingredients on the label. Some cures just sneaked in ahead of the deadline, such as this 1905 remedy, Gloria's Tonic Tablets. These uplifting-sounding pills could apparently banish rheumatism, as Mrs Jacob Sexhauer confirmed. For thirty-three years an incurable rheumatic, according to her doctors, just a few packets of Gloria's magical pills had her cured. Hot Springs Liver Buttons promised users that it would make their 'Liver all right and Bowels Regular', a combination for which anyone would be grateful. Apparently, one button taken at night guaranteed 'satisfaction in the morning'.

Opiates for the Masses

The active ingredients at the heart of many remedies were alcohol and opiates. Booze had long been used by medical practitioners – it was a handy anaesthetic during operations, for example, and was also used in lunatic asylums to quieten unruly patients. The benefits of opium were also celebrated, providing relief from pain, and being easy to administer. Physicians didn't really understand how it worked, but had noted the effects on patients from ancient times: it calmed agitation, relieved pain, soothed coughs and stopped up unruly bowels.

Opium was known as a medicine as far back as Ancient Greece. Its uses were first noted by Hippocrates who found that poppy heads soaked in water could be administered to patients with dropsy.

The physician of the notorious Roman Emperor Nero used an opium remedy, which contained sixty-two ingredients including viper's flesh.

POTIONS, PILLS AND MACHINES

Opium was already available in some Arab pharmacies by about the ninth century, and in Europe from the twelfth century. Culpeper included opium as a remedy in his 1649 *Physicall Directory*, but it was the patent era of medicines that saw the mixing of intoxicating substances into all manner of medicines. Perhaps the first opium-laced patent medicine was Dr Bate's Pacifick Pill mentioned in Dr John Jones's 1700 tract, *The Mysteries of Opium Reveal'd*. From the crazed enthusiasm of the prose it is evident that Dr Jones was far from an impartial observer when it came to the products of the poppy.

Indiscriminate use of spiked medicine for recreation rather than purely for health reasons was not unknown. In 1752 Samuel Johnson's wife Tetty died, hastened to her end by her appetite for laudanum (opium dissolved in alcohol, a common remedy at the time). One of the earliest opium-containing patent medicines was Godfrey's Cordial, a sweetened syrup recommended for use on colicky or restless infants but used far beyond. So popular did it prove that 'Godfrey's' soon became a generic name for the various drug-loaded syrups

In the seventeenth century, experimentation on animals became essential in the study of opium. In 1656 Christopher Wren broke new ground in human/canine relations when he injected his dog with opium.

Opium cures from the eighteenth century: for hysteria, steel filings mixed with wine, opium and 'hysterical water' were recommended; for piles, opium and frog-spawn water were liberally applied to the afflicted area.

203

chemists sold to the public. Another brand of choice were Dover's Powders, introduced in 1762, concocted by Thomas Dover, pupil of Thomas Sydenham (the inventor of laudanum), and known as the 'quicksilver doctor' due to the amount of mercury he prescribed to patients. Dover's Powders were initially prescribed for gout, but wider application for all sorts of ailments was soon discovered.

Barton Booth was a famous actor, renowned through London. He was also a terrible glutton. By the age of forty he was already an old man. Troubled by health problems he came across a book by Thomas Dover, 'doctor' and devoted advocate of mercury cures. Frustrated that the treatments his own doctors administered seemed to be having no effect, Booth summoned Dover. The doctor assured him that crude (liquid) mercury would cure him, and on 4 May 1733 he began his treatment. By 8 May he had swallowed an incredible 2lb of mercury. Understandably he began to complain of feeling very unwell, but still clung to the hope that this mercury course would cure him. His wife was more sceptical and called another doctor who took one look at him and recommended he should be bled, promptly drawing off 9oz of blood from his jugular and administering a dose of Sir Walter Raleigh's Cordial – a nostrum of the day. By 10 May he had deteriorated, and his scalp was blistered by the doctor to relieve his intense headache. All to no avail; by the evening he was dead. When he was opened up at autopsy the surgeon found 'the whole tract in the inside was lined with crude mercury, divided in globules about the bigness of pin's heads. The inside of the intestines . . . were as black as your hat . . . they would not endure the least straining without breaking in pieces'. Thomas Dover, meanwhile, had wisely absented himself, rightly guessing that his methods would be harshly criticised when shown the light of day.

POTIONS, PILLS AND MACHINES

In the nineteenth century opium became the product no household could do without, not least because it made an excellent babysitter. Troublesome children could be dosed up and left in a semi-comatose haze; colicky children could be soothed, teething pains were eased away, and for poor families a dose of opiate-containing medicine could hide hunger pains. A good few doses of medicine cost the same as a small bag of potatoes, and went a lot further. Karl Marx had noted that the English were 'always dosing their babies with opium', and children who were regularly fed various opium medicines were easily recognised by their thin, undernourished bodies and disproportionately large heads. Distracted parents could turn to products like Mother's Friend, or the ominously named Quietness. The leading brand was Mrs Winslow's Soothing Syrup, a sweetened opium brew, which depicted on the label a pink and chubby baby desperately grasping for the fix, which was dangled playfully above the crib by its mother. 'Depend on it, Mothers, it will give rest to yourselves and relief and health to your infants,' ran the caption below this disturbing scene.

People happily turned to dosing themselves on opium and laudanum from the local chemist, partly because industrialisation meant that fewer people had access to the countryside and traditional herbal remedies, and partly because patent medicines were cheap. With a visit to the doctor's costing a fair proportion of the weekly wages of the average working family, one-third of an ounce of laudanum cost only a fraction of this and was good for twenty-five individual doses (or a single massive one). During the 1800s adding opium and alcohol to patent medicines became more and more prevalent, and they were taken indiscriminately for ailments like bed-wetting and ingrowing toenails. Drugs and medicines were entirely unregulated in Britain until 1868. Products like J. Collis Browne's Chlorodyne, advertised as a cure for coughs, colds, colic, cramps, spasms, stomach ache, bowel pains, diarrhoea and sleeplessness, and which contained morphine, chloral hydrate and cannabis, were on sale in grocer's as well as chemist's. Opium and laudanum became the curse of the working classes as much as gin. An estimated four out of five Victorian families used opium on a regular basis.

However, by the 1880s a problem had emerged with abuse and addiction to these products, causing increasing concern.

Alert quacks, seeing that the attitude towards opium was changing, realised that the writing might well be on the wall for their existing products and swiftly set about flooding the market with cures for opium addiction or 'opiomania'. Sanatoriums sprang up offering guaranteed cures for addiction. Products like Orphine and Hopeine were touted as a surefire way of curing the addict, but were in fact little more than bottles of coloured water, often containing more opium and alcohol than the products they were supposed to replace. The death knell for quackish dope products was sounded around the turn of the century when new laws in

King George III was partial to doses of opium, and his son the Prince Regent was frequently incapacitated by a mixture of cherry brandy and laudanum.

Coleridge first became addicted to opium when he took it as a medicine in 1793 for a bad tooth. Byron too, took it for his hypochondria. Elizabeth Barrett Browning used it for back pain and heart problems.

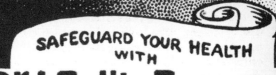
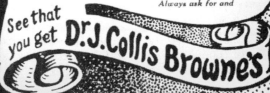

Some medicines provided a potent mixture of opium and alcohol. Ingham's Vegetable Expectorant Nervine Pain Extractor contained 86 per cent alcohol, topped off with a dash of opium. 'If sick it will do good; if well it will do no harm,' ran the pitch.

Britain, the US and France required detailed labelling of the ingredients of medicines and effectively controlled the sale of opium, heroin and cocaine.

Mrs Pinkham and her Pills

Still available today, if you know where to look, is Lydia E. Pinkham's Vegetable Compound. It was first marketed in 1875 in the back of women's magazines and journals, accompanied by testimonials from women who claimed relief from all sorts of problems after using it. It was hard being a woman, acknowledged the adverts, but Mrs Pinkham's medicine offered hope: 'A sure cure for *prolapsus uteri*, or falling of the womb and all *female weaknesses* including leucorrhoea, irregular and painful menstruation, inflammation and ulceration of the womb, flooding . . . for all weaknesses of the generative organs of either sex, it is second to no remedy that has ever been before the public, and for all diseases of the kidneys it is the *greatest remedy in the world*.'

Women were encouraged to write for advice about their medical problems to Mrs Pinkham herself, who would reply with sage recommendations usually involving the purchase of large quantities of her tonic. This ruse worked excellently until in 1905 the *Ladies Home Journal* printed a picture of Lydia's grave, revealing she had died in 1883! Denying that she had been dispensing advice from beyond the grave, the

The song 'Lily the Pink' by Liverpool band The Scaffold was a tribute to Mrs Pinkham and her pills:

We'll drink a drink a drink
To Lily the Pink the Pink the Pink
The saviour of the human race
For she invented medicinal compound
Most efficacious in every case.

company claimed that it was in fact her daughter Jennie Pinkham who had been answering the letters, a claim that was exposed as a further lie when it was revealed that a typing pool was employed to reply to the women who wrote in. However, after the 1906 law required all medicines to be labelled, it was revealed that Mrs Pinkham's medicine contained a whopping 15 per cent alcohol, stronger than most wines. For the female customers, many of whom were adamantly anti-alcohol and had taken the pledge, this was the last straw, and sales dwindled to a trickle.

H is for Cough

Around 1805, German chemist's assistant Freidrich Serturner invited some friends over to help him with a little experiment he wished to try. He had been playing around with samples of opium and had managed to extract some white crystals from it; now he wanted to see the effect they would have on humans. Somewhat cavalierly he asked his assembled guests to ingest a large quantity each, neglecting to tell them that a few days before he had accidentally killed his dog after feeding him the same substance. Almost immediately, his friends all collapsed on the floor with agonising stomach pains, vomiting and falling into profound sleep. Little did they know that they were the first people to take morphine (named after Morpheus, the Greek god of sleep), pain reliever extraordinaire, and highly addictive. Despite its shaky test run, it was welcomed by doctors as a replacement for opium and a cure for addiction to drugs and alcohol, and it was soon available for general sale and through mail order.

Morphine spawned a son, heroin, originally retailed as the safe, non-addictive alternative to morphine and opium. Heroin was the trade name the Bayer Corporation gave to this new wonder drug, and it was sold over the counter in drug kits, usually a hypodermic syringe and a phial. Marketed as a soothing remedy for chest complaints, heroin, a sovereign remedy for coughs, was available in any pharmacist.

Another drug today filed under 'recreational' is cocaine, but again this wasn't always the case. The Spaniards found that the native South Americans used coca leaf to ward off hunger and promote endurance. Initially prohibited by the conquistadores, the Spanish changed their attitude when they noticed that the local labour was a lot less productive when it wasn't chewing on coca leaves, a fact that led the Catholic Church to cultivate the crop for a while. In 1814 *Gentleman's* magazine called for research into coca, suggesting it could be used as a 'substitute for food so that people could live a month, now and then, without eating'.

In the early 1900s the philanthropic Saint James Society in the US mounted a campaign to supply free samples of heroin through the mail to morphine addicts who were trying to give up their habit.

POTIONS, PILLS AND MACHINES

Polar explorer Ernest Shackleton wandered Antarctica fuelled by tablets called 'Forced March'. An invigorating mixture of kola nut and coca leaves, each pill could 'allay hunger and prolong the power of endurance'.

Medical use of cocaine really came into its own with the isolation of its active ingredient around 1860. First used as a local anaesthetic for eye surgery, the drug soon had its biggest cheerleader in Sigmund Freud. He thought it a magical drug, and was an enthusiastic self-experimenter. Cocaine, he reasoned, could be used for a number of conditions, including digestive disorders and asthma – and as a treatment for morphine addiction.

Cocaine was soon available, like heroin, over the counter. Doctors recommended it as a cure for morphine addiction, and it found its way into a variety of patent medicines. Ryno's Hay Fever cure was 99 per cent pure cocaine 'for when the nose is stuffed up, red and sore', a nasal scenario not unlikely for regular users. Cocaine Toothache Drops proved a popular product; at 15 cents a packet they offered an instantaneous cure, although the children sedately playing on the label probably found sleep hard to come by after their nightly dose. Tonic products like coca-bola chewing gum – 'a powerful tonic to the muscular and nervous system' – and vin Mariani

Coca-laced wine proved vastly popular. Amongst it devotees were Queen Victoria, Robert Louis Stephenson, William McKinley, Alphonse XIII of Spain, assorted popes and one John Pemberton, devotee of the coca leaf and inventor of Coca-Cola.

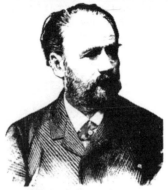

(a coca-laced wine, endorsed by the Pope and other celebrities) proved popular with consumers.

Perhaps the most famous coca product is Coca-Cola, first introduced in 1886 as a health drink – 'a valuable brain-tonic and cure for all nervous afflictions' – and an alternative to alcohol, sold in dosages of up to nine glasses per day. The drug was removed from the drink in 1903 amidst growing controversy about cocaine use, and the company ceased marketing it as a health product.

Alcohol

One group of quack products concentrated on treating drunkenness with patent medicines and concoctions. The Victorians abhorred drunkenness and quacks latched on to this market with alacrity. 'Her father was a *drunkard*,' sobbed one advert, above an illustration of a pious-looking girl. The tale of the 'plucky young lady' was related below, wherein it transpired her father had confessed after a 'spree' that he couldn't give up liquor. However, a shaft of light shone into the black despair when they discovered Antidipso, a patent cure for drunkenness,

The Civil War in America led to inordinate consumption of drugs and alcohol through patent medicines by soldiers. Hostetter's, whose brand of bitter contained 43 per cent alcohol, made 18 per cent of their turnover from sales to the forces. Addiction was so widespread it became known as 'army disease'. Peruna was one patent medicine that contained 19 per cent alcohol – sold mainly to troops, it later changed its target audience in the 1830s and was sold to women as a bust enhancer.

One doctor, L.E. Keeley, announced he had perfected a certain cure for alcoholism. This consisted of daily injections of bichloride of gold. He also gave patients a decreasing daily dose of whisky mixed with a powerful emetic, which was probably enough to put people off the drink for life. The cure became very popular and by 1892 there were eighty-two Keeley institutes in the US, with branches in Australia as well. Although the injections didn't have any therapeutic effect, Keeley's institutes did have some success in helping alcoholics give up drinking, although not in the numbers he claimed.

which the mother and daughter introduced to his meals and coffee without him knowing. After only one package, testified the young lady, her father's desire for alcohol was permanently removed, to their delight but to the chagrin of the local publican.

Most of these adverts featured attractive young women, driven to a state of hand-wringing despair by the intemperate habits of father or spouse. Women, ran the subtext, were alone capable of saving the drunkards, but only through the use of patent medicines. Unfortunately these products were near enough useless. Captain Vine Hall's Remedy for the Love of Strong Drink, for example, contained only nutmeg, peppermint and milk of magnesia.

Smoking for Health

Cigarettes and tobacco weren't always the great evil they are today. Once, not so long ago, they were considered to have useful medical applications. When the Spanish discovered tobacco in the New World they thought it was a wonder drug and enthusiastically prescribed it for all manner of things: toothache, wounds, arthritis and bad breath.

POTIONS, PILLS AND MACHINES

Smoking the right brand has always been important, like the nineteenth-century 'Cigars de Joy for Asthma and Bronchitis. One of these cigarettes gives immediate relief from the worst attack of Asthma, Hay Fever, Cough and Shortness of Breath. Their daily use effects a complete cure.' The label depicted a woman smoking her way to robust good health. In the early twentieth century, British Military HQ decided that, on the advice of doctors, soldiers should grow moustaches and smoke cigarettes to avoid infectious illness. As if being in the trenches wasn't hazardous enough.

In 1938 Dr Albert Hofman, seeking a new cure for headaches, conjured up the first LSD in his lab. Thinking the substance he had made had no use, it wasn't until the 1950s that scientists began experimenting on humans. Noted for the behavioural changes it induced in animals (researchers had even injected a three-tonne elephant with the drug), one of the first applications tried with LSD was as a cure for alcoholism. When this failed, it was given to sexually maladjusted people, schizophrenics and drug addicts in the hope they would somehow be able to view their behaviour objectively when loaded with hallucinogens, and thus 'cure' themselves. All the experiments failed, and LSD was never licensed for any therapeutic use.

Final Diagnosis

It would seem that the market and appetite for quack medicines and bizarre theories for a healthy life are, if anything, increasing. While some diseases and illnesses are in retreat as mainstream medicine advances, there is still more than enough ill health to go around. Quackery has moved its emphasis. No longer do quacks concentrate on providing a 'scientific' remedy, hoping to outwit an illiterate and ignorant public with a technical spiel beyond their comprehension. Instead they trade on the margins of lifestyle and religion. People flock to buy dubious health products on the basis of their 'natural' ingredients, like herbal drops which cure heart disease, even those 'gasping for oxygen' according to the adverts. We insist on gulping down gallons of bottled water, despite the fact that experts tell us that it is inferior to the stuff that comes from the tap. Cures which rely on some kind spiritual or psychic connection are also growing in popularity – people get pictures taken of their 'auras' with Kirlian photographs to see if they are sick, despite the fact that researchers decided any 'aura' was in fact more likely to do with the perspiration of the patient than any psychic indication of illness. Colour therapy involves patients choosing coloured jars of separated oils and shaking them up. The quicker the oils separate, the healthier the person. An oil that remains cloudy denotes a sick person, and the oils 'know' how to behave because of the energy waves projected by the patient. Some health methods skirt the edge of cultish religion, like Breatharians, who essentially believe that food is unnecessary to sustain life. All you need is good, clean air, although this wasn't enough for one follower of this health regime who was found dead from starvation in 1999. Beware the quack in all their guises.